T0362528

Hand and Upper Extremity Surgery

Editors

BRIAN W. STARR
KEVIN C. CHUNG

CLINICS IN PLASTIC SURGERY

www.plasticsurgery.theclinics.com

October 2024 • Volume 51 • Number 4

ELSEVIER

1600 John F. Kennedy Boulevard ● Suite 1800 ● Philadelphia, Pennsylvania, 19103-2899

http://www.theclinics.com

CLINICS IN PLASTIC SURGERY Volume 51, Number 4
October 2024 ISSN 0094-1298, ISBN-13: 978-0-443-13155-4

Editor: Stacy Eastman
Developmental Editor: Anita Chamoli

Clinics in Plastic Surgery (ISSN 0094-1298) is published quarterly by Elsevier Inc., 360 Park Avenue South, New York, NY 10010-1710. Months of issue are January, April, July, and October. Business and Editorial Offices: 1600 John F. Kennedy Blvd., Suite 1800, Philadelphia, PA 19103-2899. Periodicals postage paid at New York, NY and additional mailing offices. Subscription prices are $576.00 per year for US individuals, $100.00 per year for US students/residents, $631.00 per year for Canadian individuals, $703.00 per year for international individuals, $100.00 per year for Canadian students/residents, and $305.00 per year for international students/residents. For institutional access pricing please contact Customer Service via the contact information below. To receive student/resident rate, orders must be accompanied by name of affiliated institution, date of term, and the *signature* of program/residency coordinator on institution letterhead. Orders will be billed at individual rate until proof of status is received. Foreign air speed delivery is included in all *Clinics* subscription prices. All prices are subject to change without notice. Orders, claims, and journal inquiries: Please visit our Support Hub page https://service.elsevier.com for assistance.

Reprints. For copies of 100 or more of articles in this publication, please contact the Commercial Reprints Department, Elsevier Inc., 360 Park Avenue South, New York, New York 10010-1710. Tel.: +1-212-633-3874; Fax: +1-212-633-3820; E-mail: reprints@elsevier.com.

Clinics in Plastic Surgery is covered in *Current Contents, EMBASE/Excerpta Medica, Science Citation Index, MEDLINE/PubMed (Index Medicus), ASCA,* and *ISI/BIOMED.*

Contributors

EDITORS

BRIAN W. STARR, MD
Staff Surgeon, Section Pediatric Plastic and
Reconstructive Surgery, Instructor, Division of
Pediatric Plastic Surgery, Department of
Surgery, Cincinnati Children's Hospital Medical
Center, University of Cincinnati College of
Medicine, Cincinnati, Ohio, USA

KEVIN C. CHUNG, MD, MS
Professor, Department of Surgery, Chief of
Hand Surgery, Section of Plastic Surgery,
Department of Plastic Surgery, The University
of Michigan Health System, University of
Michigan Hospital, University of Michigan, Ann
Arbor, Michigan, USA

AUTHORS

UTKAN AYDIN, MD
Hand and Plastic Surgeon, Hand Surgery
Section, Department of Orthopedic Surgery
and Hand Surgery, Akademiska Hospital,
Uppsala, Sweden

JONATHAN T. BACOS, MD
Resident, Department of Plastic Surgery,
Medical College of Wisconsin, Wauwatosa,
Wisconsin, USA

CHRISTINE S.W. BEST, MD
Surgery House Officer, Department of Surgery,
Section of Plastic Surgery, University of
Michigan, Ann Arbor, Michigan, USA

RONALD D. BROWN, MD
Assistant Professor, Hand and Plastic Surgery,
Department of Plastic and Reconstructive
Surgery, The Ohio State University Hand and
Upper Extremity Center, Columbus, Ohio,
USA

TSZ KIT KEVIN CHAN, MD
Clinical Assistant Professor, Department
of Orthopedic Surgery, The University of
Michigan Health System, Ann Arbor, Michigan,
USA

MICHELE CHRISTY, MD
Resident Physician, Department of
Orthopaedic Surgery, Washington University in
St. Louis, St Louis, Missouri, USA

JOHNNY CHUIENG-YI LU, MD, MSCI
Associate Professor, Division of
Reconstructive Microsurgery, Department of
Plastic Surgery, Chang Gung University,
Chang Gung Memorial Hospital, Taoyuan,
Taiwan

KEVIN C. CHUNG, MD, MS
Professor, Department of Surgery, Chief of
Hand Surgery, Section of Plastic Surgery,
Department of Plastic Surgery, The University
of Michigan Health System, University of
Michigan Hospital, Ann Arbor, Michigan, USA

CHRISTOPHER J. DY, MD, MPH
Associate Professor, Department of
Orthopaedic Surgery, Washington University in
St. Louis, St Louis, Missouri, USA

JOHN BRADFORD HILL, MD
Assistant Professor, Department of Plastic
Surgery, Vanderbilt University Medical Center,
Nashville, Tennessee, USA

ANDREW JOSEPH JAMES, BS
Department of Plastic Surgery, Vanderbilt
University Medical Center, Nashville,
Tennessee, USA

ANTHONY M. KORDAHI, MD
Clinical Instructor, Division of Hand Surgery,
Department of Orthopedic Surgery, University
of Chicago and Biological Sciences, Chicago,
Illinois, USA

THEODORE A. KUNG, MD
Associate Professor, Department of Surgery, Section of Plastic Surgery, University of Michigan, Ann Arbor, Michigan, USA

ZHIXUE LIM, MBChB, BMedSc, MRCS
Senior Resident, Department of Hand and Reconstructive Microsurgery, National University Health System, Singapore

KEVIN J. LITTLE, MD
Professor, Director of Pediatric Hand and Upper Extremity Center, Division of Pediatric Orthopedic Surgery, Cincinnati Children's Hospital Medical Center, University of Cincinnati College of Medicine, Cincinnati, Ohio, USA

ERIN A. MILLER, MD, MS, FACS
Assistant Professor, Division of Plastic Surgery, Department of Surgery, University of Washington Medical Center, Seattle, Washington, USA

FRANCISCO DEL PIÑAL, MD, Dr Med
Private Practice, Head, Hand, Wrist and Microvascular Surgery, Madrid, Spain

SARAH E. SASOR, MD
Assistant Professor, Department of Plastic Surgery, Medical College of Wisconsin, Wauwatosa, Wisconsin, USA

SANDEEP JACOB SEBASTIN, MMed (Surgery), MCh (Plastic Surgery)
Senior Consultant, Department of Hand and Reconstructive Microsurgery, National University Health System, Singapore

ELIZABETH DALE SLATER, MD
Associate Professor, Department of Plastic Surgery, Vanderbilt University Medical Center, Nashville, Tennessee, USA

BRIAN W. STARR, MD
Staff Surgeon, Section Pediatric Plastic and Reconstructive Surgery, Instructor, Division of Pediatric Plastic Surgery, Department of Surgery, Cincinnati Children's Hospital Medical Center, University of Cincinnati College of Medicine, Cincinnati, Ohio, USA

LINDSEY TEAL, MD, MPH
Resident Physician, Division of Plastic Surgery, Department of Surgery, University of Washington Medical Center, Seattle, Washington, USA

JIGNESH V. UNADKAT, MD
Associate Professor, Division of Plastic Surgery, University of Chicago, The University of Chicago Medicine and Biological Sciences, Chicago, Illinois, USA

DEXTER W. WEEKS, MD
Hand Surgery Fellow, Department of Orthopaedic Surgery, The Ohio State University Hand and Upper Extremity Center, Columbus, Ohio, USA

SOO JIN WOO, MD
Staff, W Institute for Hand and Reconstructive Microsurgery, W General Hospital, Daegu, South Korea; Associate Professor, Division of Reconstructive Microsurgery, Department of Plastic Surgery, Chang Gung University, Chang Gung Memorial Hospital, Taoyuan, Taiwan

Contents

 Video content accompanies this article at http://www.plasticsurgery.theclinics.com.

Flexor tendon injuries require surgical repair. Early repair is optimal, but staged repair may be indicated for delayed presentations. Zone II flexor tendon injuries are the most difficult to achieve acceptable outcomes and require special attention for appropriate repair. Surgical techniques to repair flexor tendons have evolved over the past several decades and principles include core strand repair using at least a 4 strand technique, epitendinous suture to add strength and gliding properties, and pulley venting. Early postoperative active range of motion within the first 3 to 5 days of surgery is essential for optimizing outcomes.

Peripheral nerve surgeries for compressive neuropathy in the upper extremity are generally successful. However, cases that either fail or have complications requiring revision surgery are challenging. During revision consideration, surgeons should perform a comprehensive preoperative workup to understand the etiology of the patient's symptoms and categorize symptoms as persistent, recurrent, or new in relation to the index procedure. Revision surgery often requires an open, extensile approach with additional procedures to optimize outcomes. Even with proper workup and treatment, clinical outcomes of revision surgeries are inferior compared to primary surgeries and patients should be well informed prior to undergoing such procedures.

Upper extremity peripheral nerve injuries present functional deficits that are amenable to management by tendon or nerve transfers. The principles of tendon and nerve transfers are discussed, with technical descriptions of preferred tendon and nerve transfers for radial, median, and ulnar nerve injuries.

Nerve transfer surgery utilizes the redundant and synergistic innervation of intact muscle groups to rehabilitate motor function. This is achieved by transferring functional nerves or fascicles to damaged nerves near the target area, thereby reducing the reinnervation distance and time. The techniques encompass both proximal and distal nerve transfers, customized according to the specific injury. Successful nerve transfer hinges on accurate diagnosis, innovative surgical approaches, and the judicious choice of donor nerves to maximize functional restoration. This study explores nerve transfer strategies and their integration with other procedures, emphasizing their importance in enhancing outcomes in brachial plexus injury management.

There have been dwindling numbers of replantations in the United States. Despite the advocacy for centralization in hand trauma, the fundamental landscape and attitudes of surgeons toward replantation have remained lackluster. There is growing and substantial evidence to demonstrate the superior outcomes of replantation in comparison to revision amputation in most scenarios. This article aims to delve into the factors contributing to the decreasing numbers of replantations and proposes strategies to overcome this issue.

Traumatic thumb injuries significantly affect overall hand function and may result in considerable disability. Reconstructing the traumatized thumb requires a detailed preoperative assessment of the defect and evaluation of the patient's social history and medical comorbidities. Reconstructive techniques can be stratified by the level of thumb injury. The goals of thumb reconstruction are to restore length, stability, mobility, and sensibility. This article reviews reconstructive principles and operative techniques for reconstructing the traumatized thumb.

Functional impairment, absence, or traumatic loss of the thumb is associated with considerable morbidity. A fully functioning thumb is estimated to account for 40% of hand function. An array of options exists for thumb reconstruction, and the intervention selected must be tailored to each individual patient. Pollicization is a powerful and elegant operation that can dramatically improve function for many patients. However, the surgeon and patient must be keenly aware that pollicization does not construct a "normal" thumb. Herein, we present a stepwise approach to treatment, including surgical nuances, alternatives to pollicization, complications, and outcomes.

Upper extremity amputation can lead to significant functional morbidity. The main goals after amputation are to minimize pain and maintain or improve functional status while optimizing the quality of life. Postamputation pain is common and can be addressed with regenerative peripheral nerve interface surgery or targeted muscle reinnervation surgery. Both modalities are effective in treating residual limb pain and phantom limb pain, as well as improving prosthetic use. Differences in surgical technique between the 2 approaches need to be weighed when deciding what strategy may be most appropriate for the patient.

CLINICS IN PLASTIC SURGERY

SERIES OF RELATED INTEREST

Facial Plastic Surgery Clinics
https://www.facialplastic.theclinics.com/
Otolaryngologic Clinics
https://www.oto.theclinics.com/
Advances in Cosmetic Surgery
www.advancesincosmeticsurgery.com/

THE CLINICS ARE AVAILABLE ONLINE!
Access your subscription at:
www.theclinics.com

Preface
Hand and Upper-Extremity Surgery

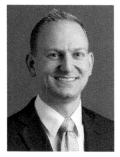 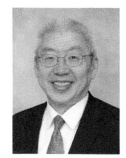

Brian W. Starr, MD   Kevin C. Chung, MD, MS

Editors

The field of hand surgery has a rich history that has evolved and expanded through the tireless contributions of countless surgeons across several specialties. In a melding of plastics, orthopedics, and general surgical principles, modern hand surgery was born out of World War II. The devastation of war created a dire need for a thoughtful, comprehensive approach to complex hand trauma. In pioneering this new frontier of subspecialized care, Sterling Bunnell acknowledged that hand surgery was a "composite problem requiring the correlation of the various specialties... the knowledge of any one of which alone is inadequate for repairing the hand."

Meticulous tissue handling, intricate reconstructive techniques, and innovative approaches to soft tissue and nerve repair have long been fundamental tenets of plastic surgery. The embrace of plastic surgery principles, coupled with an appreciation for the underlying osseous stability, biology, and biomechanics continues to push the boundaries of functional and aesthetic recovery. Today, hand surgeons continue to build on this legacy, utilizing advanced microsurgical techniques and interdisciplinary collaboration to restore function and improve the quality of life for patients with hand and upper-extremity conditions.

This *Clinics in Plastic Surgery* issue encompasses 13 meticulously curated articles that delve into the complexities and advancements in hand surgery, designed to enrich the knowledge base and practical skills of plastic and reconstructive surgeons. Each article is crafted to provide in-depth insights and up-to-date techniques in various specialized areas, reflecting the latest research and clinical practices in the field. We would like to express our sincere appreciation for our authors, who have toiled on nights and weekends—after clinics, operations, bedtimes, and family dinners—to bring this publication to life.

Brian W. Starr, MD
Section Pediatric Plastic and
Reconstructive Surgery
Cincinnati Children's Hospital
Medical Center
Department of Surgery
University of Cincinnati College
of Medicine
Cincinnati, OH 45229, USA

Kevin C. Chung, MD, MS
Department of Surgery
Section of Plastic Surgery
University of Michigan
1500 East Medical Center Drive
2130 Taubman Center, SPC 5340
Ann Arbor, MI 48109, USA

E-mail addresses:
Brian.starr@cchmc.org (B.W. Starr)
kecchung@med.umich.edu (K.C. Chung)

Clin Plastic Surg 51 (2024) ix
https://doi.org/10.1016/j.cps.2024.07.001
0094-1298/24/© 2024 Published by Elsevier Inc.

Principles for Achieving Predictable Outcomes in Flexor Tendon Repair

Erin A. Miller, MD, MS*, Lindsey Teal, MD, MPH

KEYWORDS

- Flexor tendon injury • Flexor tendon laceration • Zone II • Epitendinous repair • Core strand repair
- Pulley venting • Early active mobilization

KEY POINTS

- Flexor tendon injuries should be repaired at the earliest possible interval. Staged tendon reconstruction is indicated with delayed presentation.
- Strength of tendon repair is proportional to the number of core strands used.
- Good outcomes can be achieved with sound repair technique, regardless of surgeon preference regarding specific suture method and materials.
- Selective pulley venting is encouraged to ensure unimpeded gliding.
- Special attention to postoperative therapy is essential; early postoperative active range of motion is ideal.

 Video content accompanies this article at http://www.plasticsurgery.theclinics.com.

INTRODUCTION

Flexor tendon lacerations are commonly seen by the hand surgeon, and all require surgical repair to restore function. The ability to freely flex the digits and perform both gross and fine motor function is dependent on tendon integrity and gliding. Zone II is of particular importance as this is the most difficult area to achieve good outcomes and accounts for 24% to 50% of all flexor tendon injuries.[1,2] Historically, treatment of flexor injuries resulted in poor clinical outcomes as infection was of primary concern. Traditionally, the standard of care was to allow the wound to heal and then secondarily repair the injury by excision of the tendon and tendon grafting.[3] In the 1960s, increased prevalence of antibiotics allowed for early primary repair. Since this shift to early repair, great advances have been made in suture materials and surgical technique including epitendinous suture, multistrand core suture repair, pulley venting, and wide awake local anesthesia no tourniquet (WALANT) surgery. Advances in hand therapy including early postoperative mobilization have also improved outcomes with flexor tendon repair. While the ideal outcome is to restore finger motion to the premorbid state, this remains a difficult goal requiring meticulous technique. Achieving a predictable outcome can be simplified by following several key principles.

ANATOMY

Each finger is flexed by 2 flexor tendons: the flexor digitorum profundus (FDP) and the flexor digitorum superficialis (FDS). The FDP lies deep to the FDS in the palm, but in the digit, it courses superficial to the FDS which splits at the level of

Division of Plastic Surgery, Department of Surgery, University of Washington Medical Center, 325 9th Avenue, Seattle, WA 98104, USA
* Corresponding author.
E-mail address: erinmill@uw.edu

Clin Plastic Surg 51 (2024) 445–457
https://doi.org/10.1016/j.cps.2024.02.011

the metacarpophalangeal joint. It is important to note that lumbricals arise from the FDP tendon over the metacarpals and insert onto the radial aspect of the extensor expansion at the level of the proximal phalanx of all digits except the thumb; the presence of a lumbrical muscle on a tendon helps with its identification. The normal cascade of the fingers is in a slightly flexed position with increased flexion of the more ulnar digits; in flexor tendon injuries, the loss of integrity of the tendon causes extension of the digit and lack of tenodesis (**Fig. 1**).

The flexor tendons are held tightly against the phalanges by fibrous tendon sheaths called pulleys. The ability of the flexor tendon to efficiently contract is dependent on intact pulleys, which serve as a fulcrum for optimizing tendon flexion and extension. There are 5 annular pulleys (A1–A5) and 3 cruciate pulleys (C1–C3) on each digit (**Fig. 2**). Two pulleys of particular importance are the A2 and A4 pulleys, as these are most biomechanically advantageous to prevent bowstringing of the flexor tendon away from the phalanx.

The thumb is powered by a single flexor tendon, the flexor pollicis longus, to flex the interphalangeal (IP) joint. Given the shorter length of the thumb, the pulley system is abbreviated with A1, oblique, and A2 pulleys. Anatomically, the oblique pulley provides the most important mechanical advantage.

The flexor tendons are stratified into 5 zones-based landmarks in the volar hand (**Fig. 3**).

- Zone I: Distal to FDS insertion (fingertip to midpoint of the middle phalanx). An injury in this region would severe the FDP tendon only.
- Zone II: From the FDS insertion to proximal border of the A1 pulley (midpoint of middle phalanx to distal of palmar crease). Both the FDP and FDS run in this zone and may be injured with a sharp laceration in this location.
- Zone III: From the proximal A1 pulley to origin of lumbricals from FDP tendons (distal palmar crease to distal transverse carpal ligament). There is a high likelihood of concomitant digital nerve or artery injury with lacerations in the palm.
- Zone IV: Within the carpal tunnel beneath the transverse carpal ligament. All digital flexors lie tightly together within this zone, and multiple tendon injuries are common.
- Zone V: Proximal to the transverse carpal ligament. This zone can include muscle injuries in the forearm.

The thumb has unique zones because of its shorter length and single tendon.

- Zone TI: Distal to interphalangeal joint.

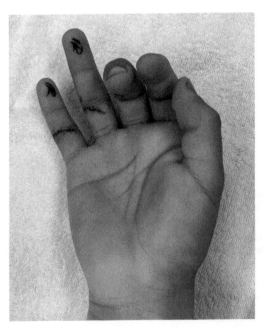

Fig. 1. Abnormal cascade of the fingers in a flexor tendon injury: note the ring and small fingers are extended relative to the adjacent digits. Lacerations are seen over zone II.

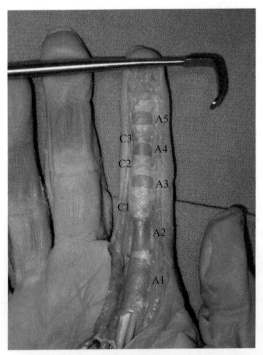

Fig. 2. Anatomy of flexor pulley system in a cadaver index finger. Five annular pulleys (A1–A5) and 3 cruciate pulleys (C1–C3) are highlighted.

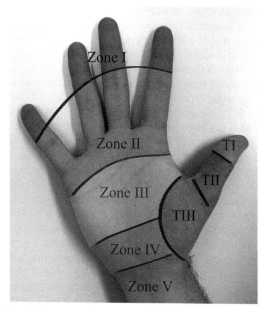

Fig. 3. Flexor tendon zones in the hand (Zones I–IV) and thumb (T1–3).

- Zone TII: Interphalangeal joint to the proximal A1 pulley.
- Zone TIII: From the thenar eminence to the transverse carpal ligament.

The surrounding environment in which a tendon lies can influence the healing capacity. Tendons surrounded by synovial sheath are classified as intrasynovial tendons, whereas tendons surrounded by subcutaneous tissue are extrasynovial tendons. Intrasynovial tendons are lubricated by synovial fluid from the surrounding epitenon, whereas extrasynovial tendons are surrounded by connective tissue called paratenon. Paratenon in extrasynovial tendons is not as proficient gliding when compared to the epitenon, but it is well vascularized and promotes wound healing. Tendons in zone I–IV area intrasynovial and transition to extrasynovial in zone V. This is important when considering healing potential, as zone V injuries heal the most reliably given the improved direct blood supply.

Although the intrasynovial tendons are primarily nourished by synovial fluid, there is additional arterial flow to the tendon from the vincula. Each flexor has 2 vincula, brevia, and longa, which lie deep to the tendon at the level of the distal interphalangeal (DIP) and base of the first phalanx, respectively. While these delicate structures may be torn with tendon retraction at the time of injury, when intact they should be preserved to improve the blood flow and healing potential.

The overall anatomy of the finger should be recalled during the evaluation of any flexor tendon injury; the neurovascular bundles run immediately adjacent to the flexor tendons along the length of the palm and into the digits. Zone II and III injuries frequently have concomitant digital nerve injuries, and the surgeon should take care to assess 2 point discrimination at the fingertip to identify additional injuries that warrant repair. With deep lacerations, the digital arteries are at risk and finger perfusion must be confirmed before proceeding to the operating theater.

PRINCIPLES OF REPAIR

The goal of tendon repair is to restore motion. Immobilization is in direct opposition to achieving this functional outcome, and the hand surgeon knows that the longer a joint or tendon is immobilized the worse the outcome. Thus, the guiding principle of tendon repair is restoring motion as soon as possible. To allow early motion, the repair must have adequate strength. In some zones, this is easy to achieve as larger, stronger sutures may be used, but in zone II, thick suture or bulky repair precludes tendon motion through the sheath and leads to inadequate motion or tendon rupture. Strength and gliding should be the primary focus of the surgeon intraoperatively, and these 2 principles are discussed at length in later zone-specific sections.

Timing of repair is paramount in the functional outcome of primary flexor tendon repair. Immediate primary repair of the flexor tendons has shown the best functional outcomes for flexor tendon excursion postoperatively.[4] Ideally, primary end-to-end repair is performed within 2 weeks of injury. When tendon repair is delayed, the retracted tendons begin to form scars and cannot be brought back out to length. Eventually, the pulley system also develops fibrosis which prevents passage of the tendon through the sheath.

In the setting of a delayed presentation greater than 2 weeks, secondary flexor tendon reconstruction is typically required in either a 1 or 2 stage tendon graft.[5] Single-stage reconstruction is more frequently performed in zone III–V injuries. If the wound bed is clean, the scarred tendon can be excised and exchanged for a free tendon graft. Donor tendons should be an appropriate size match for the excised recipient tendons, with common donor tendons being palmaris longus, plantaris, and extensor indicis proprius.[6] In zone I and II injuries, the pulley system is infrequently preserved and a 2 stage procedure is recommended. During the first stage, the flexor tendon and fibrotic tissue within the sheath are excised, and a silicone rod is placed as a spacer to form a smooth gliding surface. After an interval of no less than 3 months for the synovial sheath to form, the second stage of the surgery is performed, exchanging the rod for a free tendon graft. Full passive motion should be ensured prior to the second stage, and early motion started postoperatively to achieve the optimal outcome.

Many tendon lacerations are sharp, meaning that soft tissue coverage is adequate. In those tendon injuries with a wider zone of injury that have inadequate soft tissue coverage, a 2 stage repair is indicated. More recent knowledge in flexor tendon repair stressed the importance of minimizing incisions, as this decreases postoperative edema thus allowing earlier motion.

Postoperative therapy is as—if not more—important than the surgical procedure itself. Patient buy-in and access to a knowledgeable hand therapist are critical to success. The goals of rehabilitation are to minimize scarring and regain motion while protecting the surgical repair. A dorsal blocking splint is used to prevent uncontrolled extension that would jeopardize the repair, worn for 4 to 6 weeks postoperatively. In a robust repair, early active range of motion is initiated between days 2 to 5 postoperatively, with the aim to achieve partial active flexion and extension of digits during the first week.[7] By the end of week 3, full active flexion and extension of digits are the goal.[8] Even in situations where repair integrity or patient compliance do not allow for early active motion, passive motion protocols will still promote some tendon gliding to prevent dense adhesions. Therapy should not be neglected in any circumstance, as in adults even the most technically sound repair will not move if the digit is immobilized for several weeks postoperatively.

ZONE I INJURIES

Zone I injuries involve the FDP tendon alone as they occur distal to the FDS tendon insertion. These injuries are attributed to either a laceration of the FDP tendon or an avulsion of the tendon from its insertion on the proximal distal phalanx. A common mechanism for an avulsion injury is forced passive extension to the DIP joint while actively flexing a digit, such as grabbing another person's jersey in a sports game, leading to the term "jersey finger."[9] On examination, the patient is unable to flex the DIP joint while the PIP is held immobilized.

If there is 1 cm of length on the distal aspect of the FDP tendon for placing a core strand suture, the tendon can be primarily repaired end-to-end as described in the following section. When a small distal segment of FDP tendon remains, Wu and Tang advocate using a 10-12 strand core suture using a 4-0 permanent suture.[10] The proximal FDP is securely attached to the distal residual FDP tendon, along with periosteum at the distal insertion on the volar plate. As there is minimal to no need for tendon gliding at this distal level, bulky repair is acceptable and desirable as it will increase the strength of repair.

If the tendon is avulsed, it is typically repaired to the bone. Either suture anchors or the pull-out technique may be used; both result in similar clinical outcomes for repair of FDP tendon.[11] The pullout technique is a more traditional method used to affix the tendon to bone by placing a suture through the tendon end and passing this through the bone and dorsal soft tissues to tie over a button outside the skin.[12] The suture and button are removed after interval healing has occurred. Complications include nail bed deformity and infection.[13] Alternative technique uses a suture anchor into the distal phalanx to affix the tendon to bone, which has similar clinical outcomes with motion; the dreaded complication in this procedure is failure of the suture anchor.[11]

In repairs with a significant distal stump of FDP, these often lie in the region of the A4 pulley. Sacrifice of the A4 pulley is acceptable to achieve full visualization of the tendon ends and access for repair, given that in these injuries, the remainder of the pulley sheath is intact.

ZONE II INJURIES

Zone II flexor tendon injuries are the most difficult to treat, given the perfect fit of the tendon within the pulley system. Historically, repairs in this region were fraught complications including stiffness, ruptures, and poor outcomes, prompting surgeons to designate zone II as "no man's land." Although a bulky tendon repair yields better strength, it will not fit easily through the pulleys and precludes smooth gliding and motion. Armed with current knowledge, the surgeon can achieve reliable outcomes through careful optimization of tendon exposure, repair strength, and management of the pulley system.

Exposure

The goal of tendon exposure is to minimize the length of incisions while still able to see to evaluate and manage the tendinous injury. While a wide exposure along the length of the finger provides good working room for repair, the increased edema and soft tissue adhesions created by long incisions are detrimental to the immediate postoperative as well as the final motion achieved. Tendon ends are exposed through either Bruner or midaxial incisions. A combination of these is frequently used to incorporate the initial injury laceration. The Bruner incision, a zig-zag pattern on the volar aspect of the digit that alternates directions at the flexor creases, provides improved visualization to midline structures with less soft tissue elevation than the midaxial.[14] Both incisions protect the neurovascular bundles and prevent contractures of the volar aspect of digit. We recommend marking incisions along the entire finger for *planning purposes* so if the need to extend arises the overall pattern is appropriate, then only using the necessary length for exposure (**Fig. 4**A, B).

We advocate for adequate incision to be used for retrieval and exposure of the tendon ends to see 1 cm of tendon proximally and distally for proper suture placement with avoidance of extending further than this visualization requires. Attempting to do the repair entirely through a transverse injury laceration often leads to inadequate bites of tendon and precludes visualization of gliding to ensure the repair is not catching. It is important to note that many tendon injuries occur with the digits in flexion. This means that additional distal exposure is frequently needed to access the distal tendon stump, with the digit extended.

It is not uncommon for the proximal end of the tendon to be retracted into the palm, especially if the repair has been delayed. In these cases, the tendon must be retrieved through the pulleys prior to repair. Atraumatic retrieval techniques should be attempted to prevent adhesions that could result from an extended proximal incision. Flexion

of the wrist and metacarpal phalangeal (MCP) joints can aid in delivery of the flexor tendon; "milking" of the tendon often leads to further retraction.[15] If the tendon remains retracted in the palm, a separate 1.5 cm counter incision is made over the distal palmar crease at the affected digit as opposed to extending incisions along the length of the finger.[8] Once the tendon is visualized, it is pulled distally with a fine hemostat and then passed through the flexor tendon sheath. While many surgeons are taught to use a tendon passer, this is frequently too bulky to fit through a long length of the sheath. We find that flexible tubing, such as a suction catheter or pediatric feeding tube, passes easily through the flexor tendon sheath; once the tubing is retrieved in the palm, the tendon is sutured to it and the tubing used to pull the tendon back into its native position in the sheath.[16] The tendon may be secured proximally with a 25 gauge needle through the proximal sheath to atraumatically hold it off tension while the repair is performed (**Fig. 4**C). The digit should be kept flexed to maximize tendon length during repair.

Flexor Digitorum Superficialis Management

At the level of the A2 pulley over the proximal phalanx, the FDS courses volar to the FDP tendon at the proximal aspect of the A2 pulley, and then splits into a radial and ulnar slips at the distal aspect of the A2 pulley and allows the FDP to then course volar to the FDP slips. It is important during retrieval that the FDP is not twisted around the FDS, as this will increase friction and consequently stress on the

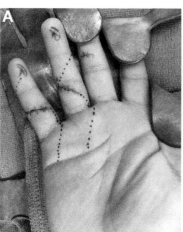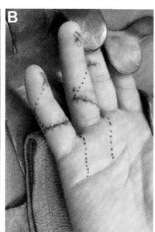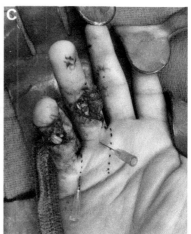

Fig. 4. (*A*) Planning of Bruner incisions along volar aspect of digits. (*B*) For the small finger, the initial laceration is not conducive to a Bruner incision and thus a combination of Bruner and midaxial incisions are planned. (*C*) Demonstration of conservative use of incisions: the entire Bruner is avoided and only additional length necessary for exposure is used. The proximal aspects of the tendons were delivered into the wound underneath the A2 pulley using a fine hemostat and were held in place using a 25 gauge needle.

repair. With a complete laceration of both tendons, the surgeon must decide whether to repair one slip, both slips, or not repair the FDS at all. While some would argue for repair of both slips of the FDS to restore normal anatomy, the bulk of the repair in addition to the FDP repair frequently leads to crowding within the A2 pulley, impairing gliding ability and increasing stress on the repair. Therefore, within the A2 pulley, many surgeons opt to only repair FDP or repair FDP and one slip of FDS.[3,8,17,18] We advocate evaluation of patient factors in this decision; in patients who may have a more challenging time with rehab, FDP only repair is our preference. In compliant patients, we choose to only repair one slip of the FDS, as the crowding effect of 3 suture repairs within the proximal pulley system is significant enough to worsen outcomes (Fig. 5).

Repair Sutures

Epitendinous repair is a circumferential repair along the periphery of the tendon that has been shown to further increase the strength of the repair and improve the gliding ability of the tendon by creating a smoother surface along the tendon.[19,20] The epintendinous repair is typically performed with 6 to 0 prolene in a simple running manner.[21] The peripheral suture is placed in the epitenon 2 mm from the tendon edge at the repair site.[22] Although many surgeons use an epitendinous repair once the tendon has been fixed, epitendinous suture placement prior to core suture repair in zone II injuries has shown a 20% increase in repair strength and decreased tendinous gliding resistance.[23,24] We find that placing the back wall epitendinous suture first helps align the tendon for core suture repair, yielding a less bulky repair overall (Fig. 6A, B).

One of the major advancements in surgical techniques over the past several decades is the improved strength of flexor tendon repair using core suture techniques. The strength of the repair is dependent on suture choice, the length of core suture purchase, the suture technique, and most importantly the number of strands spanning the repair.[20]

Selecting the appropriate caliber of suture is a balance between strength and gliding function. Although larger sutures result in increased tensile strength, sutures larger than a 3 to 0 are bulky and can impede tendon gliding[25,26]; 3-0 or 4-0 caliber sutures should be used. The type of suture used should be nonabsorbable, have high tensile strength, and minimal bulk. Stainless steel and Fiberwire, while high in tensile strength, result in bulky knots. Prolene, nylon, and Ethibond have

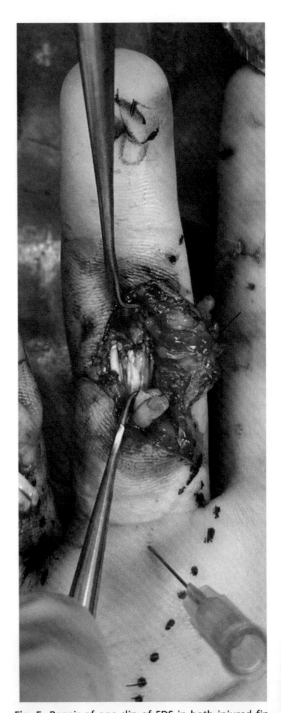

Fig. 5. Repair of one slip of FDS in both injured fingers. A core figure of 8 suture is used and then a 6 to 0 prolene epitendinous to smooth the anterior wall and promote gliding of the subsequent FDP repair.

lower but adequate tensile strength and are less bulky with knot formation; however, these monofilament sutures may have slippage.[27] We prefer a braided polyamide suture (Supramid) for the high

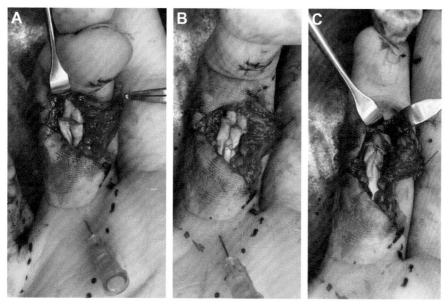

Fig. 6. FDP repair. (*A*) Placement of the back wall of the epitendinous suture first ensures that the flexor tendon is well aligned and off tension during placement of the core suture. (*B*) Core suture in place: a looped 4 to 0 Supramid was used in a cruciate pattern. Note bites of the tendon are 10 mm back from the cut edge. (*C*) The epitendinous suture is completed along the front wall to smooth the repair to improve gliding.

tensile strength and increased friction creating tendon grasping properties.

Regardless of suture pattern, the optimal suture purchase from the tendon edge is between 0.7 and 1 cm, with suture purchase of 0.4 cm or less resulting in much weaker repair.[28] Looped sutures may be used, as they provide double the number of core strands across the tendon without further damaging the tissue or increasing the number of knots. Suture technique also varies in whether it is locking or grasping. Locking sutures wrap around the tendon fibers and prevent suture sliding through the tendon when tensioned; grasping sutures also increase tensile strength by increasing friction but to a lesser degree as they pull through tendon fibers when tensioned. Both locking and grasping techniques increase tensile strength to varying degrees.[29] Care should be taken with locking sutures, however, as they cannot be further tensioned when the knot is tied; the appropriate tension on the repair must be maintained throughout placement, making the repair technically difficult. While grasping or nonlocking sutures have the ability to be tensioned once placed in the tendon, care must be taken to not pull toward the cut edge to avoid sutures pull through toward the cut tendon end and decreasing the purchase.

The strength of the core suture repair is directly related to the number of strands that pass the repair site.[30] To create adequate strength for early active motion, a minimum of 4 strands is required.

The 6 strand repair results in a firmer repair with less pliability and gapping.[31] Clinical outcomes comparing the 4 and 6 strand repairs have demonstrated similar grip strength, with the 6 strand repair superior in total active motion (TAM).[32] Eight or more strand repairs are also used by experienced surgeons when a stronger repair is needed.[33] A variety of suture patterns may be used to achieve adequate number of strands crossing the repair; commonly used are the Kessler and modified Kessler—these are 2 strand repairs that require an additional suture (typically a horizontal mattress) to be placed to create a 4 strand repair. This creates extrabulk with the addition of a second knot. Common 4 strand core repair techniques include the double Kessler and the cruciate techniques. The M-Tang technique is a straightforward, 6 strand core repair technique, with excellent reported outcomes, performed with looped suture (**Fig. 7**).[34] Each of these suture techniques can be modified to use grasping or locking bites based on the surgeon's preference (see **Fig. 6**B).

Tension across the repair is important to prevent gapping in the tendon during digit flexion. A gap across the repair means that tendon ends are no longer in contact and cannot heal, thus rupture happens when the suture is stressed at physiologic loads. Maintaining tendon contact is paramount to healing. Increasing the tension on the suture results in bulkiness of the tendon at the repair site and

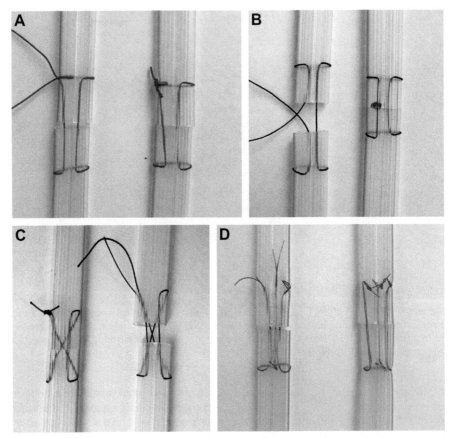

Fig. 7. Core suture patterns. (*A*) Kessler: this 2 strand repair needs to be supplemented with a horizontal mattress to create a repair of adequate strength for early active motion. (*B*) Modified Kessler: note the knot is in the repair site. (*C*) Cruciate repair places 4 strands across the repair site with 1 knot. (*D*) M-tang repair creates a 6 strand repair.

helps to prevent gapping that may happen as the tendon flattens during physiologic loading. Repairs should ideally be tensioned 10-20% bulky, as during repetitive motion cycles the sutures settle into the tendon leading to separation at the repair site which may cause gapping in non-bulky repairs.[31]

Given the critical importance of ongoing tendon contact for healing, the investigators wish to identify gapping at the time of repair. We take the finger through 20 to 30 cycles of motion once the repair is complete, applying significant stress across the repair by straightening the finger to full extension, to ensure the sutures have settled and identify if any gapping is present. If the repair gaps with cycles, it is revised.

Pulley Management

Once the tendon repair is complete, range of motion is assessed intraoperatively (Video 1). This ensures that there is no tendinous gapping with extension of the digit and that the flexor tendon glides easily.[31,35] If there is resistance to gliding between the tendon and the pulley, it must be addressed. Given the goal of a bulky repair, the tendon is larger than the pulley, and if during excursion it must pass through a pulley there is often resistance or frank catching of the repair (especially when both tendons are repaired). To alleviate this, pulleys are vented during repair for unrestricted gliding. The typical distance of tendon gliding with full range of motion is 1.5 to 2 cm; therefore, less than 2 cm of the pulley sheath needs to be released for adequate gliding.[31]

Biomechanically, the A2 and A4 pulleys are critical to maintaining full excursion of the finger.[36] Previous doctrine that the A2 and A4 pulleys must remain intact to prevent bowstringing has been challenged in recent years, and the current evidence supports the ability to regain full excursion with complete release of either A2 or A4 provided the other pulleys remain intact.[37] The pulleys are vented longitudinally several millimeters at a time and the range of motion tested until the repair no longe catches. In the thumb, while the oblique pulley is most critical in prevention of bowstringing, it may be sacrificed if both A1 and A2 are intact (**Fig. 8**).

Although we do not support indiscriminate pulley release, we find that final motion is improved with more aggressive release and do not hesitate to fully vent either A2 or A4 if the repair appears

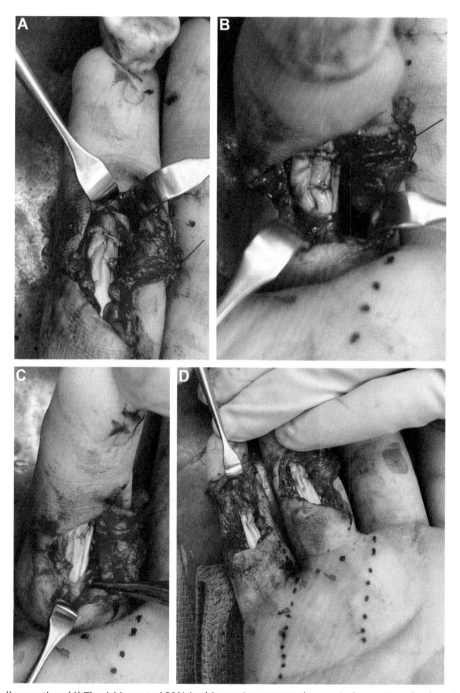

Fig. 8. Pulley venting. (*A*) The A4 is vented 30% in this repair to ensure the repair does not catch when the finger is fully straightened. (*B*) The A2 is evaluated; with the finger flexed, the tendon is not passing smoothly through the repair as evidenced by the tendon appearing to be loose distally. (*C*) The A2 is vented 30% and the tension on the tendon normalizes. (*D*) The finger is cycled through range of motion to ensure no gapping at full extension and confirm adequate gliding of the tendons.

to catch at these sites. Even some mild bowstringing will provide a better outcome than a tendon repair which ruptures because it cannot pass through the pulley, so when in question, we err on the side of release.

Rehabilitation

Postoperatively, the upper extremity is placed in a dorsal blocking splint to prevent finger extension which causes tension across the repair. The splint spans from the distal forearm to the tips of the digits with the wrist in a neutral position, the MCP joints in flexion, and the IP joints in slight flexion.[7] Early mobilization within 3 to 5 days of surgery facilitates a functional recovery. Both active and passive range of motion protocols have good functional outcomes; while we prefer early active range of motion, the more critical aspect is the comfort of the hand therapist with the protocol and the ability of the patient to comply. Full active flexion of the digits begins in the sixth postoperative week, when the repair has gained strength.

ZONE III–V INJURIES

Repairing flexor tendons in zones III, IV, and V is less technically demanding than repairs in zones I and II. Tendons in zones III–V are extrasynovial and surrounded by connective tissue that aids in wound healing and gliding. Given the proximity of the tendons in zones III–V to nerves and vessels, concomitant injury is common. Standard core suture repairs in these zones should be implemented with at least a 4 strand repair. The goal in the proximal zones is strength, and these repairs may be bulky as they do not have a tight tunnel through which they must glide. Zone IV encompasses the carpal tunnel, and therefore the transverse carpal ligament is released as part of the exposure. Zone IV and V flexor tendon injuries almost always involve multiple tendons, and each structure should be visualized to ensure no injury is missed. Owing to concomitant neurovascular injuries in this zone, early rehabilitation is often impaired.[38] Given the ability to add strength with a bulkier repair and the lack of increased tension created by the pulley system, these repairs are less prone to rupture and can be rehabilitated more aggressively with good outcomes.

COMPLICATIONS

Flexor tendon repair is a balancing act. On the one side, we have the complication of stiffness, and on the other we find tendon rupture; both adhesions and rupture occur at a rate of 4%.[39] Stiffness often occurs secondary to adhesion formation along the wound bed. Adhesions impair tendon gliding and excursion and may be treated with tenolysis. Tenolysis is a reasonable consideration in the compliant patient who reaches a plateau in hand therapy, with a passive arc of motion that surpasses active motion. Full passive flexion must be present prior to undertaking tenolysis.[40] Surgery is ideally performed wide awake to continuously assess active motion and to ensure that all adhesions are released.[41] After flexor tendon tenolysis, 80% of patients show improvement of symptoms. However, appropriate patient selection and counseling are critical, as flexor tendon rupture rates are reported in up to 16% of patients.[42,43]

Tendinous rupture falls on the other end of the spectrum of complications of flexor tendon repair. If the rupture occurs early within the postoperative period, early re-exploration and primary repair within a few days are indicated. In those tendons that were rerepaired within 72 hours of the initial repair, over 50% achieved good or excellent results with a rerupture rate of 12.5%.[44] If the rupture occurs later, staged reconstruction is indicated with a flexor tendon graft. A silicone rod is placed at the time of rupture followed by a staged secondary procedure with a tendon graft.[25]

OUTCOMES

A retrospective multicenter cohort study published by Tobler-Ammann and colleagues evaluated the outcomes of 218 patients who underwent repair of zone I–III flexor tendon injuries at 1 year postoperatively. Range of motion was assessed by measuring the TAM score and the ability of the digit to touch the palm. The function was measured using the disability of the arm shoulder and hand (DASH) questionnaire. Patients in the study underwent early active range of motion and all had at least a 4 strand core suture repair. They found a rupture rate of 8.7% and good to excellent return of motion. Patient's functional outcomes measured by the DASH questionnaire were found to be significantly improved in all outcomes except pain at 26 weeks, which showed improvement up to 13 weeks postoperatively.[45]

A meta-analysis done by Xu and colleagues assessed the outcomes of 569 digits that underwent repair of zone II flexor digit injuries. The analysis compared the rates of tendon rupture and range of motion, measured by TAM score, between patients who underwent early active range of motion and those who underwent early passive range of motion with the Kleinert and Duran protocols. They found greater range of motion in patients who underwent early active range of motion compared to early passive range of motion (good to excellent results in 50% in early passive range of motion group and 94% in early active range of motion group). A significantly higher rate of flexor tendon rupture was found in those who underwent early active range of motion compared to early passive range of motion. On subgroup analysis, increased rupture with early active motion was found only in groups who underwent 2 strand core suture techniques. No difference in rupture rate was found in tendons repaired with at least a 4 strand core suture technique.[46]

A randomized prospective trial done by Trumble and colleagues evaluated the outcomes of 119 digits that underwent zone II flexor tendon repair. Tendons were repaired using a 4 strand core suture technique with epitendinous repair. The patients were randomized into either early active or early passive range of motion protocol. Outcomes measured included interphalangeal joint range of motion, dexterity tests, DASH score, flexion contracture, and patient satisfaction. The early active range of motion group had greater range of motion, increased patient satisfaction, and decreased rates of flexion contracture. The DASH score and dexterity tests had no significant difference between the 2 groups.[47]

ACHIEVING RELIABLE OUTCOMES

Outcomes in flexor tendon repair vary greatly and are partly dependent on patient participation in post-op therapies. The surgeon can optimize the potential for a full recovery in a compliant patient by adhering to the following principles. The author's specific approach to zone II tendon repair is as follows:

- *Patient education* regarding the injury and need for postoperative therapy beginning at the preoperative visit.
- *Early repair*, ideally within the first 2 weeks to ensure primary repair possible.
- *Limiting incisions* to only what is required for adequate visualization: counter incisions in the palm are recommended for proximal tendon retrieval instead of further extending incisions along the finger (see **Fig. 4**).
- Adequate *strength of repair to allow for early active motion*—a minimum of 4 strands. Looped sutures may be used to increase the strength. We strongly recommend epitendinous suture both for the additional tensile strength and smoothing tendon contour allowing for better gliding (**Figs. 5–7**).
- Intraoperative testing of repair by taking the finger from flexion to full extension to ensure

no gapping: repair should be redone if tendon ends lose contact (see Video 1).
- Critical evaluation of tendon gliding through the pulleys: repair of only one slip of FDS to increase space (with excision of the other slip) and *venting of pulleys* if any concern. Pulleys should be released to the extent needed that the repair passes without resistance; either A2 or A4 should be fully maintained (see **Fig. 8**).
- *Therapy should start 3 to 5 days postoperatively* with a certified hand therapist; while early active motion protocols have superior outcomes, we have found that therapist comfort with the regimen is more critical than the exact protocol.

SUMMARY

Flexor tendon injuries, specifically zone II, are common in hand trauma, and the treatment has continued to evolve over the past several decades. Flexor tendon injuries should be surgically repaired early, if possible. Staged tendon reconstruction is often necessary with delayed presentation. Key surgical points include minimizing incisions, using at least a 4 strand core repair technique, and judicious pulley venting to allow for adequate strength and tendon gliding. Early postoperative active range of motion is essential for optimal recovery and results in improved overall range of motion.

CLINICS CARE POINTS

- Patient education and expectation setting for proper rehabilitation should begin at the preoperative visit.
- Tendon repair should be performed at the earliest possible interval, ideally within 1 week.
- Incisions should be limited by employing counter incisions rather than extensions to retrieve proximal tendon stumps.
- Repair should be of appropriate strength using at least 4 core strands, performed in a slightly bulky manner, to facilitate early active motion.
- Venting of the pulley system, including A2 OR A4 to ensure gliding of the repair.
- Intraoperative testing to confirm smooth gliding and no gapping at the repair site.
- Early initiation of postoperative therapy within 3 to 5 days.

DISCLOSURE

The authors have no relevant disclosures to report.

SUPPLEMENTARY DATA

Supplementary data to this article can be found online at https://doi.org/10.1016/j.cps.2024.02.011.

REFERENCES

1. de Jong JP, Nguyen JT, Sonnema AJ, et al. The incidence of acute traumatic tendon injuries in the hand and wrist: a 10-year population-based study. Clin Orthop Surg 2014;6(2):196–202.

2. Ranjan V, Mehta M, Mehta M, et al. The outcomes of flexor tendon injury repair of the hand: a clinico-epidemiological study. Cureus 2023;15(1):e33912.

3. Kotwal PP, Ansari MT. Zone 2 flexor tendon injuries: venturing into the no man's land. Indian J Orthop 2012;46(6):608–15.

4. Tang J, Shi D, Gu Y. [Flexor tendon repair: timing of surgery and sheath management]. Zhonghua Wai Ke Za Zhi [Chinese Journal of Surgery] 1995;33(9):532–5.

5. Strickland JW. Delayed treatment of flexor tendon injuries including grafting. Hand Clin 2005;21(2):219–43.

6. Battiston B, Triolo PF, Bernardi A, et al. Secondary repair of flexor tendon injuries. Injury 2013;44(3):340–5.

7. Tang JB. Rehabilitation after flexor tendon repair and others: a safe and efficient protocol. J Hand Surg Eur 2021;46(8):813–7.

8. Tang JB. Flexor tendon injuries. Clin Plast Surg 2019;46(3):295–306.

9. Leddy JP, Packer JW. Avulsion of the profundus tendon insertion in athletes. J Hand Surg Am 1977;2(1):66–9.

10. Wu YF, Tang JB. Letter regarding "a 10- or 12-strand core suture in a flexor tendon in zones I, II, and III". J Hand Surg Am 2015;40(12):2510–1.

11. McCallister WV, Ambrose HC, Katolik LI, et al. Comparison of pullout button versus suture anchor for zone I flexor tendon repair. J Hand Surg Am 2006;31(2):246–51.

12. Azarpira M, Asmar G, Falcone MO. Modified pull-out technique for zone one flexor digitorum profundus repair. Arch Bone Jt Surg 2022;10(11):976–81.

13. Kang N, Marsh D, Dewar D. The morbidity of the button-over-nail technique for zone 1 flexor tendon repairs. Should we still be using this technique? J Hand Surg Eur 2008;33(5):566–70.

14. Bruner JM. Surgical exposure of flexor tendons in the hand. Ann R Coll Surg Engl 1973;53(2):84–94.

15. Griffin M, Hindocha S, Jordan D, et al. An overview of the management of flexor tendon injuries. Open Orthop J 2012;6:28–35.

16. Ozturk MB, Basat SO, Kayadibi T, et al. Atraumatic Flexor tendon retrieval- a simple method. Ann Surg Innov Res 2013;7(1):11.

17. Elliot D, Giesen T. Primary flexor tendon surgery: the search for a perfect result. Hand Clin 2013;29(2):191–206.

18. Henry M. Zone II: repair or resect the flexor digitorum superficialis? J Hand Surg Am 2011;36(6):1073–5.

19. Wieskötter B, Herbort M, Langer M, et al. The impact of different peripheral suture techniques on the biomechanical stability in flexor tendon repair. Arch Orthop Trauma Surg 2018;138(1):139–45.

20. Wu YF, Tang JB. Recent developments in flexor tendon repair techniques and factors influencing strength of the tendon repair. J Hand Surg Eur 2014;39(1):6–19.

21. Shalimar A, Lim CH, Wong SK, et al. A survey of zone II flexor tendon repair techniques and rehabilitation protocols preferred by Malaysian orthopaedic practitioners. Malays Orthop J 2022;16(2):87–94.

22. Merrell GA, Wolfe SW, Kacena WJ, et al. The effect of increased peripheral suture purchase on the strength of flexor tendon repairs. J Hand Surg Am 2003;28(3):464–8.

23. Galvez MG, Comer GC, Chattopadhyay A, et al. Gliding resistance after epitendinous-first repair of flexor digitorum profundus in zone II. J Hand Surg Am 2017;42(8):662. e1-e9.

24. Papandrea R, Seitz WH Jr, Shapiro P, et al. Biomechanical and clinical evaluation of the epitenon-first technique of flexor tendon repair. J Hand Surg Am 1995;20(2):261–6.

25. Elliot D, Giesen T. Treatment of unfavourable results of flexor tendon surgery: ruptured repairs, tethered repairs and pulley incompetence. Indian J Plast Surg 2013;46(3):458–71.

26. Taras JS, Raphael JS, Marczyk SC, et al. Evaluation of suture caliber in flexor tendon repair. J Hand Surg Am 2001;26(6):1100–4.

27. Rudge WBJ, James M. Flexor tendon injuries in the hand: a UK survey of repair techniques and suture materials—are we following the evidence? ISRN Plastic Surgery 2014;2014:1–4.

28. Tang JB, Zhang Y, Cao Y, et al. Core suture purchase affects strength of tendon repairs. J Hand Surg Am 2005;30(6):1262–6.

29. Hotokezaka S, Manske PR. Differences between locking loops and grasping loops: effects on 2-strand core suture. J Hand Surg Am 1997;22(6):995–1003.

30. Savage R, Risitano G. Flexor tendon repair using a "six strand" method of repair and early active mobilisation. J Hand Surg Br 1989;14(4):396–9.

31. Tang JB. New developments are improving flexor tendon repair. Plast Reconstr Surg 2018;141(6):1427–37.

32. Sadek A, Nourelden A, Elshwikh A, et al. Four-strands versus six-strands core sutures technique for surgical management of acute zone II flexor tendon injury. Minia Journal of Medical Research 2020;31(3):291–7.

33. Lee HI, Lee JS, Kim TH, et al. Comparison of flexor tendon suture techniques including 1 using 10 strands. J Hand Surg Am 2015;40(7):1369–76.

34. Tang JB, Pan ZJ, Munz G, et al. Flexor tendon repair techniques: m-tang repair. Hand Clin 2023;39(2): 141–9.

35. Fulchignoni C, Alessandri Bonetti M, Rovere G, et al. Wide awake surgery for flexor tendon primary repair: a literature review. Orthop Rev 2020;12(Suppl 1): 8668.

36. Chow JC, Sensinger J, McNeal D, et al. Importance of proximal A2 and A4 pulleys to maintaining kinematics in the hand: a biomechanical study. Hand (N Y) 2014;9(1):105–11.

37. Moriya K, Yoshizu T, Tsubokawa N, et al. Clinical results of releasing the entire A2 pulley after flexor tendon repair in zone 2C. J Hand Surg Eur 2016; 41(8):822–8.

38. Klifto CS, Capo JT, Sapienza A, et al. Flexor tendon injuries. J Am Acad Orthop Surg 2018;26(2):e26–35.

39. Dy CJ, Hernandez-Soria A, Ma Y, et al. Complications after flexor tendon repair: a systematic review and meta-analysis. J Hand Surg Am 2012;37(3): 543–51.e1.

40. Wu KY, Gillis JA, Moran SL. Secondary procedures following flexor tendon reconstruction. Plast Reconstr Surg 2022;149(1):108e–20e.

41. Lalonde DH, Martin AL. Wide-awake flexor tendon repair and early tendon mobilization in zones 1 and 2. Hand Clin 2013;29(2):207–13.

42. Whitaker JH, Strickland JW, Ellis RK. The role of flexor tenolysis in the palm and digits. J Hand Surg Am 1977;2(6):462–70.

43. Eggli S, Dietsche A, Eggli S, et al. Tenolysis after combined digital injuries in zone II. Ann Plast Surg 2005;55(3):266–71.

44. Dowd MB, Figus A, Harris SB, et al. The results of immediate re-repair of zone 1 and 2 primary flexor tendon repairs which rupture. J Hand Surg Br 2006;31(5):507–13.

45. Tobler-Ammann B, Beckmann-Fries V, Calcagni M, et al. Outcomes of 218 primary single-finger flexor tendon repairs up to 1 year after surgery: a multicentre cohort study. J Hand Surg Eur 2023;48(9): 911–9.

46. Xu H, Huang X, Guo Z, et al. Outcome of surgical repair and rehabilitation of flexor tendon injuries in zone II of the hand: systematic review and meta-analysis. J Hand Surg Am 2023;48(4):407. e1-e11.

47. Trumble TE, Vedder NB, Seiler JG 3rd, et al. Zone-II flexor tendon repair: a randomized prospective trial of active place-and-hold therapy compared with passive motion therapy. J Bone Joint Surg Am 2010;92(6):1381–9.

Optimizing Outcomes in Revision Peripheral Nerve Surgery of the Upper Extremity

Michele Christy, MD, Christopher J. Dy, MD, MPH*

KEYWORDS

- Revision peripheral nerve surgery • Carpal tunnel syndrome • Cubital tunnel syndrome
- Nerve compression

KEY POINTS

- In patients requiring revision peripheral nerve surgery, surgeons should categorize symptoms as recurrent, persistent, or new to narrow the differential diagnoses and help build a surgical plan.
- The most likely etiology requiring revision carpal tunnel surgery is incomplete release of the median nerve in which case the authors recommend open decompression and external neurolysis to identify healthy median nerve both proximally and distally to the site of injury.
- Open decompression and external neurolysis alone are often insufficient in cases of revision cubital tunnel syndrome, and the authors prefer to add submuscular transposition of the ulnar nerve to optimize its course about the elbow.
- Given a lack of strong supporting evidence, the authors do not currently use any of the commercially available barriers for revision ulnar or median nerve surgery and prefer autologous local adipofascial tissue.

INTRODUCTION

Peripheral nerve pathology of the upper extremity is common and can have a significant impact on an individual's function and quality of life.[1–4] Patients with peripheral nerve injury often present with complaints of intermittent, burning-type pain, numbness, and paresthesias in a focal distribution. Carpal tunnel syndrome (CTS), a specific peripheral nerve pathology, is the most common entrapment neuropathy with an estimated prevalence rate of 1% to 5% of the general population.[5–8] Consequently, carpal tunnel release, the treatment of choice for CTS, is the most frequently performed hand procedure. Although carpal tunnel release often has favorable results, a complication and/or failure rate of 1% to 25% has been reported in the literature with 1% to 12% of patients requiring secondary surgery.[9–14] Patients considered to have failed primary carpal tunnel release include those with no improvement in symptoms 12 months postoperatively or those with initial improvement in symptoms followed by clinical deterioration.[12] Similar failure statistics are reported for cubital tunnel syndrome (CuTS), the second most common compression neuropathy of the upper extremity.[15–18]

Patients with CTS and CuTS who fail initial treatment are considered for revision surgery. In the revision setting, regardless of the nerve or location of pathology, it is helpful to categorize patients into 1 of 3 groups: persistent, recurrent, or new symptoms.[10] Patients with persistent symptoms fail to experience significant relief from the initial procedure and continue to have pain of the same quality and distribution as prior to surgery. Patients categorized as "recurrent" experience a temporary resolution of symptoms postoperatively before

Department of Orthopaedic Surgery, Washington University in St. Louis, 660 South Euclid Avenue, Campus Box 8233, St Louis, MO 63110, USA
* Corresponding author. 660 South Euclid Avenue, Campus Box 8233, St Louis, MO 63110.
E-mail address: Dyc@wustl.edu

Clin Plastic Surg 51 (2024) 459–472
https://doi.org/10.1016/j.cps.2024.02.012
0094-1298/24/© 2024 Elsevier Inc. All rights reserved.

return of symptoms. When assessing these patients, it is critical to evaluate whether the patient's symptoms are identical to what they experienced prior to their index surgery or different.[1,10] Finally, patients may experience "new" complaints after their initial procedure.[10,13] The most common etiology of new symptoms are iatrogenic from surgery or from a secondary pathology that may or may not be related to the initial procedure.[6,10]

When evaluating patients who have experienced failure of their primary procedure, it is important to perform a comprehensive clinical workup and consider various surgical techniques to plan for revision surgery. Through the lens of CTS and CuTS, this article will discuss key steps in preoperative, intraoperative, and postoperative management of patients with recalcitrant nerve symptoms to optimize outcomes of revision intervention.

PERSISTENT, RECURRENT, OR WORSENING SYMPTOMS AFTER CARPAL TUNNEL RELEASE
Etiology

The most common cause of persistent CTS is from incomplete decompression of the median nerve.[19] This often occurs from inadequate release of the transverse carpal ligament distally or antebrachial fascia proximally (**Fig. 1**), most commonly due to insufficient surgical exposure and visualization.[10,13,20,21] Further, symptoms may persist due to secondary sites of median nerve compression in the forearm. Common secondary sites of compression are between the 2 heads of the pronator teres, the flexor digitorum superficialis (FDS) arch (**Fig. 2**), the ligament of Struthers and/or the lacertus fibrosus.[22–24] There is also a well-documented relationship between patients with CTS and cervico-brachialgia.[25] Eason and colleagues detailed that in patients who reported suboptimal results after carpal tunnel decompression, 81% of them had additional complaints of neck pain and/or abnormal cervical spine radiographs prior to their carpal tunnel release. This double crush phenomenon is important to consider in the revision peripheral nerve setting because it has been shown that patients with double crush syndrome have lower satisfaction scores and worse outcomes after peripheral nerve surgery regardless of cervical spine intervention.[26]

Secondary sites of compression can cause persistent symptoms as well as manifest as a recurrence of symptoms several months postoperatively.[6,10] However, when a patient is complaining of a recurrence of symptoms, it is most commonly due to tethering of the nerve from scar formation, especially when the incision is

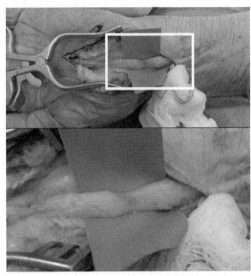

Fig. 1. Top and bottom photos demonstrate intraoperative findings of the median nerve during revision carpal tunnel surgery after incomplete primary release of the distal antebrachial fascia and proximal component of the flexor retinaculum. This image was captured after both longitudinal and transverse epineural neurolysis was completed and demonstrates significant bruising, narrowing, and flattening at the compression site with median nerve swelling both proximally and distally. (*Courtesy of* Christopher J Dy, MD, MPH; used with permission.)

placed directly over the median nerve.[10,27] Surgical factors that can contribute to increased scar formation include prolonged postoperative immobilization, inadequate hemostasis leading to hematoma formation, and/or insufficient hand therapy.[10] Additional preoperative risk factors that have been associated with revision surgery include male sex, tobacco use, rheumatoid arthritis, and bilateral CTS.[14]

Finally, new symptoms are often the result of iatrogenic injury to the median nerve, ulnar nerve or

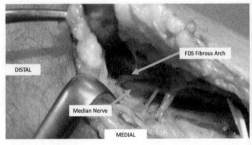

Fig. 2. Intraoperative example of proximal median nerve compression as it passes deep to a distinct fibrous FDS arch. (*Courtesy of* Christopher J Dy, MD MPH; used with permission.)

their branches (**Fig. 3**).[28–31] The palmar cutaneous branch of the median nerve is most commonly injured and is at greater risk with radially curved thenar incisions.[32,33] Additionally, the terminal branch of the median nerve that supplies the third webspace is prone to injury at the distal aspect of the surgical release. These injuries as well as additional pathologies including piso-triquetral pain syndrome, carpal arch alterations, and flexor tendon bowstringing should be considered in patients with new symptoms following carpal tunnel decompression.[34–37]

Clinical Evaluation

A comprehensive history and full musculoskeletal neurovascular examination should be performed in all cases of recalcitrant CTS. The history should elicit timing, quality, location, and severity of symptoms, which helps stratify patients into 1 of the 3 aforementioned categories. The standard physical examination as well as provocative maneuvers can help further narrow the differential diagnoses.[38,39] Positive Durkan and/or Phalen tests are suggestive of continued pathology within the carpal tunnel.[40,41] Tinel test can be performed throughout the upper extremity to help localize the site of injury. Importantly, the test will elicit a positive response 2 to 4 inches proximal to the actual area of injury.[10,41] Gainor compression test evaluates median nerve compression more proximally in the forearm and is positive with tenderness over the pronator teres or with forearm pain aggravated by resisted pronation or middle finger FDS contraction.[42,43] Sensory changes over the thenar eminence is also suggestive of pronator syndrome because the palmar cutaneous branch of the median nerve is often affected due to compression proximal to its branching.

High-resolution ultrasonography is a cost-effective, noninvasive tool that can be used to identify the precise location, type of lesion, and extent of peripheral nerve injury.[44–46] Ultrasound has been proven to be both sensitive and specific for diagnosing peripheral nerve injury in both the acute and revision settings.[47–49] Duetzmnn and colleagues evaluated 116 patients prior to undergoing revision carpal tunnel surgery and found that a cross-sectional area cutoff of 14.5 mm^2 was 78% sensitive and 97% specific in diagnosing ongoing or recurrent CTS.[48]

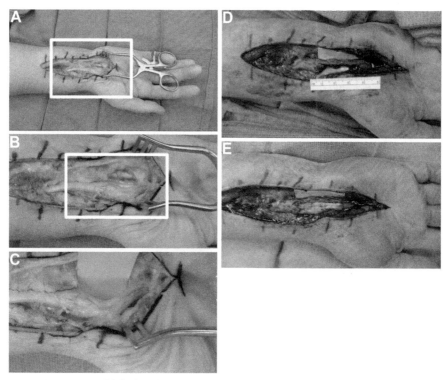

Fig. 3. Intraoperative images of failed median nerve decompression due to nerve injury. (*A–C*) The median nerve has been exposed during a revision procedure and is found to course through dense scar tissue with associated tethering to the radial side of the incision. *White boxes* in *A* and *B* delineate the zoomed in area in *C*. (*D*) Internal and external neurolysis was performed. The zone of injury was identified and the neuroma was resected until there was healthy median nerve both proximally and distally. (*E*) Autograft was used to repair the defect. (*Courtesy of* Christopher J Dy, MD, MPH; used with permission.)

Electrodiagnostic (EDX) studies are another helpful preoperative tool, especially if the clinical examination elicits symptoms that are vague or can be explained by multiple pathologies. When considering revision peripheral nerve surgery, it is helpful to compare an updated EDX to prior examinations. A sudden significant change in motor or sensory nerve function suggests acute nerve injury.[50–52] Though the degree of nerve conduction velocity slowing and presence of secondary axonal changes can help gauge the severity of nerve injury, this information is unlikely to impact the type of revisional procedure that is performed.[23,53] It is also important to recognize that EDX findings will not return to normal after a prior decompression, even if the patient has experienced complete symptom resolution.

While the authors do not routinely obtain MRI as part of the clinical workup in the revision peripheral nerve setting, literature does support its use in identifying incomplete nerve release and recurrent nerve compression due to scar formation.[54–56] In a study by Taghizadeh and colleagues, they found that MRI was accurate in identifying incomplete release or regrowth of the transverse carpal ligament following carpal tunnel release, but it was unhelpful when trying to perform an accurate quantitative assessment of the transverse carpal ligament.[55]

Another intervention that is reported but not routinely used by the authors is a steroid injection into the carpal tunnel. Beck and colleagues suggest that a steroid injection into the carpal tunnel can be used as a preoperative indicator of how patients will respond to revision carpal tunnel decompression.[57] While their results were not statistically significant, they did suggest that results from a cortisone injection predicted the outcome of revision carpal tunnel release 87% of the time.

Management

Once the surgeon understands the likely etiology of symptoms, a candid, 2-way discussion regarding the risks, benefits, and expected outcomes of revision surgery should be discussed with the patient. Contrary to the primary procedure, the authors typically prefer an extensile approach in the revision setting under general anesthesia, as opposed to local. One exception to this preference is patients with recurrence of symptoms after many years of initial symptom relief. In this situation, repeat CTR can be typically performed under local anesthesia. While carpal tunnel release has a high success rate, revision procedures are less successful. It is imperative

to inform the patient of this by setting clear preoperative expectations.[58]

Revision decompression of carpal tunnel

The authors prefer an extensile, open approach when performing revision carpal tunnel decompression. We recommend having a low threshold to extend the prior incision proximally across the wrist (in a Bruner zig-zag manner, aiming ulnarly to minimize the risk of injury to the palmar cutaneous branch of the median nerve) into the forearm to identify healthy median nerve. We then track the median nerve distally through the prior surgical site and ensure sufficient decompression. An evaluation for additional causes of nerve compression including synovitis of adjacent flexor tendons or ganglion cysts within the carpal tunnel is performed.[59] Although the authors primarily perform an open decompression for recalcitrant CTS, the literature suggests that endoscopic carpal tunnel release is an option in revision cases.[60,61] However, given the abnormal anatomy and history of failed procedure, the authors feel they are best able to ensure complete decompression via an open approach.

External and internal neurolysis

Once the median nerve is identified, external and internal neurolysis are commonly performed to remove perineural and intraneural fibrosis.[6,62] Neurolysis is complete when healthy nerve is seen intraoperatively, which can be marked by visualization of fascicles and bands of Fontana (**Fig. 4**).[6,10] Bands of Fontana are spiral appearing dark and light strips on the surface of unstretched nerves due to the structure of nerve fibers within the epineural sheath.[63] The purpose of the neurolysis is to remove scar tissue and allow for improved nerve gliding.

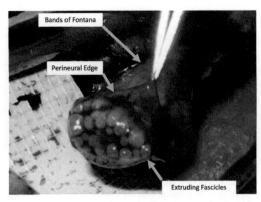

Fig. 4. Intraoperative visualization of healthy, extruding fascicles and Bands of Fontana. (*Courtesy of* Christopher J Dy, MD, MPH; used with permission.)

External neurolysis has been well studied and proven effective, especially in cases of recurrent symptoms.[64–66] While it has been shown that neurolysis is not beneficial in primary carpal tunnel decompression,[67,68] external neurolysis is performed in most cases of revision open decompression.[69] Internal neurolysis has also been proven to be safe,[70,71] and when needed, the authors use this technique to visualize normal nerve. When performing internal neurolysis, surgeons should be cautious to not disrupt the perineurium as that is part of the blood–nerve barrier. The extent of which neurolysis is performed depends on the amount of scaring and fibrosis of each nerve.[10]

Nerve coverage

There are several described vascularized and non-vascularized coverage options to insulate the median nerve when performing revision decompression. The hypothenar fat pad flap (HTFPF) is a popular surgical technique to create a barrier between the median nerve and overlying tissues to prevent recurrent scar formation and fibrosis.[72,73] This technique mobilizes a pedicled fat pad off the ulnar artery that is then transposed to the volar aspect of the median nerve, deep to the transverse carpal ligament.[72,74] In a recent meta-analysis evaluating outcomes of revision carpal tunnel decompression, Soltani and colleagues found that decompression with flap coverage was superior to decompression alone.[69] Further, the HTFPF technique improves pain, numbness, and paresthesia in patients with refractory symptoms[75] and demonstrates improvement on the Boston Carpal Tunnel Questionnaire symptom severity and functional status scale.[76]

In additional to the HTFPF, other vascularized, local tissue techniques have been described for median nerve coverage including the lumbricals,[77] abductor digiti minimi,[78] pronator quadratus,[79] palmaris brevis,[80] reverse radial artery fascial flap (Fig. 5),[81] and pedicled tenosynovial tissue flap.[82] While all of these procedures have been proven effective, there are no randomized controlled trials comparing one outcome to another. Therefore, when choosing which local soft tissue procedure to perform, the authors recommend the surgeon perform whichever procedure they are most comfortable and familiar with. In rare cases, free flap procedures have been described, but the authors would only consider one of these techniques if there are no local flap options available.[13,83–85]

There are also nonvascularized, autologous and commercial products that can be used to wrap the median nerve and prevent perineural scaring. Py and colleagues reviewed several of these

options including bovine collagen (NeuraWrap - Integra Lifesciences - Princeton, NJ, USA), procine small intestine submucosa (AxoGuard - Axogen - Tampa, FL, USA), and hyaluronic acid-carboxycellulose membrane (Seprafilm - Baxter International - Deerfield, IL, USA)[86] and concluded that there is promise in the efficacy of these barrier options, but more laboratory and clinical data are needed before adopting it to clinical practice.[86] Because of this lack of evidence, we do not recommend the use of commercial barriers in this setting.

Despite these numerous techniques and procedures, the literature is mixed regarding how much surgery should be done to try to optimize outcomes in revision cases. A recent systematic review by de Roo and colleagues suggests that there is no clinical benefit in adding additional procedures, such as soft tissue flaps or nerve wraps, to revision carpal tunnel cases when compared to decompression and neurolysis alone. Given this, the authors prefer to perform an external neurolysis and open decompression on all recalcitrant carpal tunnel cases with the addition of pedicled adipofascial flap transfer when clinically indicated (see Fig. 5).

PERSISTENT, RECURRENT, OR WORSENING SYMPTOMS AFTER CUBITAL TUNNEL SURGERY
Etiology

CuTS encompasses the symptoms caused by irritation and compression of the ulnar nerve at the elbow. The success of in situ ulnar nerve decompression, especially in patients with idiopathic CuTS, is high with the majority of patients experiencing a resolution of symptoms.[87–89] However, several preoperative risk factors have been identified as predictors of needing future revision surgery. These include younger age (<50 years old), prior elbow fracture, and performing surgery on mild clinically graded disease.[88,89]

Similar to CTS, recalcitrant CuTS can be broken down into persistent, recurrent, and/or new symptoms. There are several sites where the ulnar nerve can be compressed including the Arcade of Struthers, the medial intermuscular septum, the medial epicondyle, the cubital tunnel, and the deep aponeurosis of the flexor carpi ulnaris.[90] Persistent symptoms following primary cubital tunnel decompression can be caused by incomplete decompression, continued ulnar nerve subluxation, or a missed secondary diagnosis.[91–93] Additional pathologies such as ulnar tunnel syndrome, thoracic outlet syndrome, and/or cervical radiculopathy can present similar to CuTS and would not be addressed with cubital tunnel

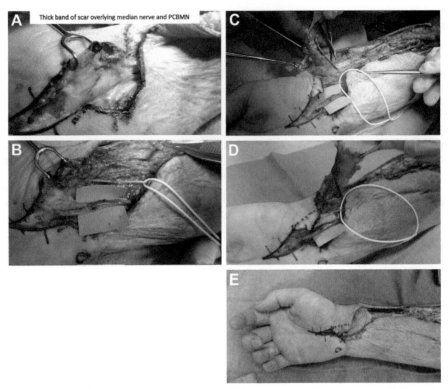

Thick band of scar overlying median nerve and PCBMN

Fig. 5. Revision CTR with radial artery perforator-based adipofascial flap. (*A*) Intraoperative image of revision CTR with extensile approach. The curvilinear incision at the base of the palm is extended across the wrist crease in a Bruner zig-zag manner. (*B*) Scar was released after identifying the radial artery, palmar cutaneous branch of the median nerve (PCBMN) and while protecting median nerve. (*C, D*) Radial artery perforator-based adipofascial flap was isolated from the distal radial and volar forearm and was rotated to cover the narrowed section of median nerve. (*E*) The adipofascial flap was rotated and inset easily and was then covered with split thickness skin graft harvested from the ipsilateral arm. (*Courtesy of* Christopher J Dy, MD, MPH; used with permission.)

decompression.[92] Of these various causes of persistent symptoms, incomplete decompression is the most common and is likely the source in up to 20% of failed cubital tunnel procedures.[87]

A period of temporary relief followed by return of symptoms after cubital tunnel surgery is most likely due to fibrosis and scar formation at the surgical site causing recurrent compression.[62] If the primary surgery included nerve transposition, new sites of compression or new instability can be a cause of recurrent pain.[94] Mackinnon and Novak reported surgical findings of 100 reoperations for CuTS and found that 55 patients had distal kinking of the ulnar nerve between the 2 heads of the flexor carpi ulnaris from its new course traveling anterior to the medial epicondyle.[94] Additionally, anterior transposition without release of the Arcade of Struthers or medial intermuscular septum can result in persistent compression at these more proximal locations.[95]

Finally, iatrogenic injury is the most common cause of new symptoms after surgery. The medial antebrachial cutaneous nerve (MABCN) commonly runs within 40 mm of the medial epicondyle and is the most vulnerable structure during cubital tunnel surgery.[91,96,97] In the aforementioned study by Mackinnon and Novak, 73 of 100 patients who underwent revision cubital tunnel surgery were found to have a neuroma of the MABCN (**Fig. 6**).[94]

Regardless of the cause of recalcitrant symptoms, it is important to have an honest conversation with patients regarding expectations before

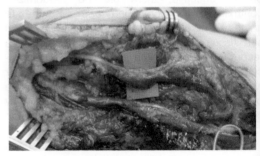

Fig. 6. Intraoperative neuroma of the MABCN during revision surgery for CuTS. (*Courtesy of* Christopher J Dy, MD, MPH; used with permission.)

undergoing revision surgery. Aleem and colleagues demonstrated that revision surgery for CuTS has good outcomes with improvement in symptoms in 79% of patients. However, revision patients have worse outcomes and are more likely to experience persistent symptoms and diminished pinch strength compared to patients who only underwent primary surgery for CuTS.[98]

Clinical Evaluation

As with the workup for CTS, a detailed history to understand the quality, timing, and severity of symptoms is important in cases of recalcitrant CuTS. Additionally, given the numerous possible sites of compression of the ulnar nerve around the elbow, it is helpful to obtain an operative report to understand the extent of primary surgery that was performed. Specific aspects of the history and physical examination can help differentiate ulnar nerve compression at the elbow versus similar pathologies. Medial elbow pain radiating down the ulnar side of the forearm and hand, weak grip, and loss of fine motor control are all suggestive of CuTS. If sensation is intact over the dorsal-ulnar hand, ulnar tunnel syndrome is more likely as the dorsal cutaneous branch of the ulnar nerve branches proximal to Guyon's canal and thus is preserved. Physical examination of the cervical spine, shoulder girdle, axilla, and supraclavicular region should be performed to assess for cervical radiculopathy, brachial plexopathy, and/or thoracic outlet syndrome. A history of cervical disc herniation has been identified as a risk factor for recalcitrant CuTS.[99]

Various provocative tests can be performed to differentiate among upper extremity pathologies. Sustained elbow flexion for 1 minute that recreates or exacerbates symptoms is suggestive of CuTS. When assessing the ulnar nerve at the cubital tunnel, it is important to palpate the nerve with both passive and active elbow flexion/extension to observe for ulnar nerve instability and subluxation. Snapping triceps can be confused with ulnar nerve subluxation at the elbow but would not be associated with the neuropathic complaints of ulnar nerve compression. Further, the nerve commonly subluxes at 90° of flexion while the triceps dislocates closer to 110°.[100] Tinel's sign is another commonly used technique that should be performed at both the medial elbow and ulnar wrist to assess for CuTS and ulnar tunnel syndrome, respectively. Davidge and colleagues described the hierarchical scratch collapse test, which was shown to accurately identify both primary and secondary sites of ulnar nerve compression.[101] In the hierarchical test, the primary site of compression is

identified and then "frozen out" with ethyl chloride as additional sites are subsequently tested.[101] Despite enthusiasm for the scratch collapse test, we have found it difficult to reliably perform, and similar information can be obtained from other aspects of the physical examination. Spurling and Lhermitte maneuvers can be used to assess cervical spine pathology, and Wright and Adson maneuvers are suggestive of thoracic outlet syndrome.[102]

As opposed to recalcitrant CTS, the role of advanced imaging and EDX studies for CuTS is less clear. Boers and colleagues demonstrated that the sensitivity of both ultrasound and EDX in cases of persistent and/or recurrent CuTS is low.[103] However, ultrasound can be used to identify postoperative anatomy, sites of adhesions, and instability of the ulnar nerve.[103] Given the lack of evidence to support the use of these advanced modalities, the authors rely heavily on their clinical findings and reserve additional tests for cases that are unclear or require testing to rule out additional pathology.

Management

Repeat decompression
In revision cubital tunnel decompression, the prior surgical scar is extended both proximally and distally. The procedure can be performed using a regional brachial plexus block and proximal fascial block for the intercostobrachial nerve, terminal medial brachial cutaneous nerve, and MABCN. However, given the extensive nature of these procedures, the authors prefer general anesthesia, which also enables the ability for the surgical team to assess the patient's clinical examination after surgery. External neurolysis is performed until normal ulnar nerve is identified both proximally and distally. The surgeon should dissect the ulnar nerve in a proximal to distal direction to help prevent inadvertently damaging any branching nerves. In revision cases, the neurolysis should be completed across the entire elbow from the medial intermuscular septum proximally to the 2 heads of the flexor carpi ulnaris distally.[91] Additionally, Gabel and Amadio assert that there are frequently at least 2 sites of ulnar nerve compression in revision cases, further emphasizing the need for wide exposure.[90] Careful investigation and identification of any neuromas should be performed. Once neurolysis is thought to be complete, the elbow should be ranged to ensure there are no remaining sites of tethering of the ulnar nerve.

In cases of recalcitrant CuTS, it is uncommon to perform open decompression and neurolysis alone.[18] It is thought that neurolysis alone will lead to recurrent tethering/adhesions and ultimately, recurrent pain. While Dagregorio and Saint-Cast demonstrated that simple neurolysis alone provided good to fair results in 8 of 9 patients at 2 year follow-up after undergoing revision surgery for CuTS,[104] it is the author's preference to perform a submuscular transposition in nearly all revision cases to minimize the chances of subsequent surgery.

Nerve transposition

There are 2 types of ulnar nerve transpositions—submuscular and subcutaneous. Submuscular ulnar nerve transposition is performed by releasing the flexor-pronator mass, transposing the nerve deep to this well-vascularized muscle bundle and repairing the muscle.[92,105,106] This has historically been the favored procedure in cases of recurrent CuTS demonstrating an average improvement in symptoms in 62% of cases.[107]

Despite historic popularity of submuscular transposition, recent studies have demonstrated noninferior outcomes with subcutaneous transposition.[108,109] Caputo and Watson published good or excellent results in 75% of patients who underwent subcutaneous transposition after failed primary surgery for CuTS.[108] In order to secure the transposed nerve, it was originally described to free fascia from the flexor-pronator origin and suture the fascia over the transposed ulnar nerve.[110] Critics of this method argue that the fascial flap does not provide an adequate environment for the nerve and can lead to recurrent perineural scaring or form a new site of compression. Another more recent trend is to utilize a pedicled adipofascial flap from perforators of the brachial artery. Theoretically, this provides a vascularized adipose bed that is thought to reduce adherence and allow for superior nerve gliding.[111,112] While this type of subcutaneous transposition is preferred by the authors for patients being treated surgically for the first time for an unstable, but electrodiagnostically healthy ulnar nerve, the authors will utilize a submuscular transposition for nearly all patients undergoing a second ulnar nerve surgery. One exception would be patients undergoing capsular contracture release for elbow stiffness. In these cases, a subcutaneous transposition is used to minimize the chances of joint effusion or recurrent capsular contracture affecting the ulnar nerve.

Nerve wrapping

As previously described with regards to recurrent CTS, numerous types of materials can be used to wrap the ulnar nerve and provide an adequate environment for nerve gliding while also reducing the risk of fibrosis and adhesions. Gasper and colleagues[113] reported 8 patients who had at least 2 failed prior ulnar nerve operations that underwent revision neurolysis and amniotic membrane wrapping. In this review, all 8 patients demonstrated improvement in visual analog scale pain levels; disabilities of the arm, shoulder and hand scores; and grip strength. Further, all 8 patients were subjectively satisfied with their results at 30 months of follow-up.[113] The saphenous vein has also been shown to be an effective adhesion barrier in cases of recalcitrant CuTS.[18,114] In a study by Kokkalis and colleagues, all 17 patients who underwent vein wrapping experienced significant pain relief and improvement in 2 point discrimination. However, they did experience transient pain and swelling in their leg from graft harvest that is not experienced in other nerve wrap options.[114] Porcine extracellular matrix has also been described with favorable results.[115] However, the authors do not use any of the current commercially available barriers for revision ulnar nerve surgery and prefer using autologous local adipofascial tissue.

Medial epicondylectomy

A medial epicondylectomy can be performed in either primary or revision cubital tunnel decompression with the intent of optimizing the course of the ulnar nerve at the medial elbow. This procedure eliminates the risk of ulnar nerve subluxation and reduces the risk of secondary sites of compression as the nerve can travel in a congruent path. There is no consensus about when it is optimal to utilize this technique. In their review titled "The Management of Failed Cubital Tunnel Decompression," Burahee and colleagues favored medial epicondylectomy over ulnar nerve transposition in revision cases.[91] Papatheodorou and colleagues also reported 12 cases of recurrent CuTS that were treated with decompression, minimal medial epicondylectomy (if not previously performed), and nerve wrapping (porcine extracellular matrix) and found significant improvement in postoperative pain, pinch strength, and grip strength.[115]

Distal nerve transfer

When managing recalcitrant and severe CuTS, revision surgery should address pain, but surgeons should also consider ways to optimize patient function. In patients with severe intrinsic muscle wasting from chronic compression of the ulnar nerve, revision decompression and neurolysis surgeries alone are unlikely to significantly improve motor function. In this subset of patients

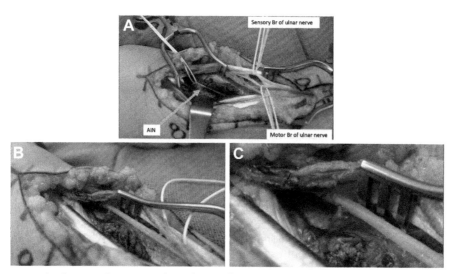

Fig. 7. Intraoperative images of reverse end to side transfer to optimize intrinsic hand motor function. (*A*) Dissection through the skin and subcutaneous tissues to find the ulnar neurovascular bundle. The superficial sensory branch of the ulnar nerve and deep motor branch were distinguished with the motor branch traveling deep to the hypothenar fascia. The hypothenar fascia was released. AIN was also identified traveling into the pronator quadratus. (*B, C*) The proximal two-thirds of the pronator quadratus was divided to further dissect out AIN, which was then divided distally. A reverse end to side nerve transfer of AIN into the motor component of the ulnar nerve was performed with nylon sutures and augmented with fibrin glue. (*Courtesy of* Christopher J Dy, MD, MPH; used with permission.)

with motor denervation on EDX, supercharged end-to-side (SETS) surgery has been described to try to optimize motor recovery.[116,117] In this technique, the neuromuscular bundle of the anterior interosseous nerve (AIN) is transposed, and coaptation with the motor unit of the ulnar nerve in the forearm is performed (**Fig. 7**).[116] Several studies have demonstrated promise in restoring at least partial intrinsic hand function in this cohort with severe disease.[117–120] While support for this technique continues to grow, the authors believe that patient selection is critical to obtaining satisfactory results. Following the guidelines of Power and colleagues, patients with decreased compound muscle action potentials on EDX studies and an adequate donor AIN can be considered for this technique.[121]

POSTOPERATIVE PREFERENCES

For both primary and revision peripheral nerve cases, the authors emphasize the importance of early mobilization to allow gliding of the nerve itself and the surrounding tissues. For cases in which nerve coaptations are not performed, we prefer starting motion of adjacent joints within 3 days of surgery. If nerve coaptations are performed, the adjacent joints are immobilized for 3 weeks; after weeks, active motion is encouraged, but passive

motion that may stretch the coaptation (such as wrist extension for a median nerve reconstruction) is limited until 6 weeks after surgery.

SUMMARY

Compressive neuropathy of the upper extremity is a relatively common musculoskeletal pathology that has excellent nonoperative and operative treatment options. However, when surgical management for these conditions fail, the surgeon is faced with a challenging problem. When considering revision surgery, it is helpful to categorize the patient's symptoms into persistent, recurrent, or new in relation to the index procedure. A comprehensive history, physical examination, and supplementary tests can be used to better understand the most likely etiology of symptoms and failure of the index procedure. For the median nerve, incomplete release is the most common etiology requiring revision surgery. For these cases, an open and extensile approach to the median nerve is preferred by extending the original incision in a Bruner zig-zag manner into the forearm to visualize healthy median nerve both proximally and distally to the site of compression. External neurolysis should be performed in all revision cases with the addition of internal neurolysis and adipofascial flap coverage when clinically indicated. For CuTS, it is helpful to understand all procedures that were performed in the index surgery to have a better idea of what additional procedures may be required in the revision setting. There is less published literature to support the use of advanced imaging and testing in the preoperative setting for revision CuTS compared to CTS. Similar to CTS, the authors recommend an extensile approach for revision CuTS with dissection in a proximal to distal direction to minimize injury to any branching neurovascular structures. The authors prefer performing submuscular transposition into addition to decompression and neurolysis in nearly all cases of revision CuTS to optimize the course of the ulnar nerve about the elbow. Given limited published evidence, the authors do not use any of the commercially available barrier options at this time and prefer using autologous local adipofascial tissue. Prior to undergoing revision surgery, all patients should be counseled on risks and probable results in order to manage expectations and optimize outcomes of revision peripheral nerve surgery in the upper extremity.

CLINICS CARE POINTS

- Neurolysis does not improve outcomes in primary carpal tunnel release but is effective and should be performed in revision cases.

- There are numerous local soft-tissue options for median nerve coverage that have all been proven to be effective with no head-to-head studies suggesting superiority of one method over another.

- There is a lack of laboratory and clinical evidence to support the use of commercial nerve barrier options at this time.

- In revision cubital tunnel decompression, neurolysis should be completed across the entire elbow from the medial intermuscular septum proximally to the 2 heads of the flexor carpi ulnaris distally with the assessment for multiple sites of ulnar nerve compression.

- Despite historic popularity of submuscular transposition of the ulnar nerve, subcutaneous transposition has been shown to have noninferior results.

- In the appropriate patient population with severe intrinsic muscle wasting from chronic compression of the ulnar nerve, SETS surgery should be considered to optimize motor recovery of the hand.

DISCLOSURE

The authors have no conflicts of interest to disclose.

REFERENCES

1. Dibbs RP, Ali K, Sarrami SM, et al. Revision peripheral nerve surgery of the upper extremity. Semin Plast Surg 2021;35(2):119–29.
2. Silver S, Ledford CC, Vogel KJ, et al. Peripheral nerve entrapment and injury in the upper extremity. Am Fam Physician 2021;103(5):275–85.
3. Miranda GE, Torres RY. Epidemiology of traumatic peripheral nerve injuries evaluated with electrodiagnostic studies in a tertiary care Hospital clinic. P R Health Sci J 2016;35(2):76–80.
4. Grinsell D, Keating CP. Peripheral nerve reconstruction after injury: a review of clinical and experimental therapies. BioMed Res Int 2014;2014: 698256.
5. Papanicolaou GD, McCabe SJ, Firrell J. The prevalence and characteristics of nerve compression symptoms in the general population. J Hand Surg Am 2001;26(3):460–6.
6. Pripotnev S, Mackinnon SE. Revision of carpal tunnel surgery. J Clin Med 2022;(5):11.
7. Gelfman R, Melton LJ 3rd, Yawn BP, et al. Long-term trends in carpal tunnel syndrome. Neurology 2009;72(1):33–41.
8. Fajardo M, Kim SH, Szabo RM. Incidence of carpal tunnel release: trends and implications within the United States ambulatory care setting. J Hand Surg Am 2012;37(8):1599–605.
9. Atroshi I, Gummesson C, Johnsson R, et al. Prevalence of carpal tunnel syndrome in a general population. JAMA 1999;282(2):153–8.
10. Tung THH, Mackinnon SE. In: Luchetti R, Amadio P, editors. Secondary carpal tunnel surgery. Carpal tunnel syndrome. . Springer; 2001. p. 307–18.
11. Neuhaus V, Christoforou D, Cheriyan T, et al. Evaluation and treatment of failed carpal tunnel release. Orthop Clin North Am 2012;43(4):439–47.
12. Karl JW, Gancarczyk SM, Strauch RJ. Complications of carpal tunnel release. Orthop Clin North Am 2016;47(2):425–33.
13. Jones NF, Ahn HC, Eo S. Revision surgery for persistent and recurrent carpal tunnel syndrome and for failed carpal tunnel release. Plast Reconstr Surg 2012;129(3):683–92.
14. Westenberg RF, Oflazoglu K, de Planque CA, et al. Revision carpal tunnel release: risk factors and rate of secondary surgery. Plast Reconstr Surg 2020; 145(5):1204–14.
15. Grandizio LC, Maschke S, Evans PJ. The management of persistent and recurrent cubital tunnel syndrome. J Hand Surg Am 2018;43(10):933–40.

16. Bartels RH, Grotenhuis JA. Anterior submuscular transposition of the ulnar nerve. For post-operative focal neuropathy at the elbow. J Bone Joint Surg Br 2004;86(7):998–1001.

17. Zlowodzki M, Chan S, Bhandari M, et al. Anterior transposition compared with simple decompression for treatment of cubital tunnel syndrome. A meta-analysis of randomized, controlled trials. J Bone Joint Surg Am 2007;89(12):2591–8.

18. Kholinne E, Alsharidah MM, Almutair O, et al. Revision surgery for refractory cubital tunnel syndrome: a systematic review. Orthop Traumatol Surg Res 2019;105(5):867–76.

19. Stutz N, Gohritz A, van Schoonhoven J, et al. Revision surgery after carpal tunnel release–analysis of the pathology in 200 cases during a 2 year period. J Hand Surg Br 2006;31(1):68–71.

20. Langloh ND, Linscheid RL. Recurrent and unrelieved carpal-tunnel syndrome. Clin Orthop Relat Res 1972;83:41–7.

21. Patrick J. Carpal tunnel syndrome. Br Med J 1965; 1(5446):1377–8.

22. Adler JA, Wolf JM. Proximal median nerve compression: pronator syndrome. J Hand Surg Am 2020;45(12):1157–65.

23. Lee DH, Claussen GC, Oh S. Clinical nerve conduction and needle electromyography studies. J Am Acad Orthop Surg 2004;12(4):276–87.

24. El-Haj M, Ding W, Sharma K, et al. Median nerve compression in the forearm: a clinical diagnosis. Hand (N Y) 2021;16(5):586–91.

25. Eason SYB RJ, Greene TL. Carpal tunnel release: analysis of suboptimal results. J Hand Surg Br 1985;10-B(3):365–9.

26. Wessel LE, Fufa DT, Canham RB, et al. Outcomes following peripheral nerve decompression with and without associated double crush syndrome: a case control study. Plast Reconstr Surg 2017; 139(1):119–27.

27. Zieske L, Ebersole GC, Davidge K, et al. Revision carpal tunnel surgery: a 10-year review of intraoperative findings and outcomes. J Hand Surg Am 2013;38(8):1530–9.

28. Conolly WB. Pitfalls in carpal tunnel decompression. Aust N Z J Surg 1978;48(4):421–5.

29. Louis DS, Greene TL, Noellert RC. Complications of carpal tunnel surgery. J Neurosurg 1985;62(3):352–6.

30. MacDonald RI, Lichtman DM, Hanlon JJ, et al. Complications of surgical release for carpal tunnel syndrome. J Hand Surg Am 1978;3(1):70–6.

31. Cartotto RC, McCabe S, Mackinnon SE. Two devastating complications of carpal tunnel surgery. Ann Plast Surg 1992;28(5):472–4.

32. Watchmaker GP, Weber D, Mackinnon SE. Avoidance of transection of the palmar cutaneous branch of the median nerve in carpal tunnel release. J Hand Surg Am 1996;21(4):644–50.

33. Taleisnik J. The palmar cutaneous branch of the median nerve and the approach to the carpal tunnel. An anatomical study. J Bone Joint Surg Am 1973;55(6):1212–7.

34. Inglis AE. Two unusual operative complications in the carpal-tunnel syndrome. A report of two cases. J Bone Joint Surg Am 1980;62(7):1208–9.

35. Seradge H, Seradge E. Piso-triquetral pain syndrome after carpal tunnel release. J Hand Surg Am 1989;14(5):858–62.

36. Gartsman GM, Kovach JC, Crouch CC, et al. Carpal arch alteration after carpal tunnel release. J Hand Surg Am 1986;11(3):372–4.

37. Bloem JJ, Pradjarahardja MC, Vuursteen PJ. The post-carpal tunnel syndrome. Causes and prevention. Neth J Surg 1986;38(2):52–5.

38. Mackinnon SE, Novak CB, Landau WM. Clinical diagnosis of carpal tunnel syndrome. JAMA 2000; 284(15):1924–5 [author reply 1925-6].

39. Wiesman IM, Novak CB, Mackinnon SE, et al. Sensitivity and specificity of clinical testing for carpal tunnel syndrome. Can J Plast Surgmer 2003; 11(2):70–2.

40. Durkan JA. A new diagnostic test for carpal tunnel syndrome. J Bone Joint Surg Am 1991;73(4):535–8.

41. Kuschner SH, Ebramzadeh E, Johnson D, et al. Tinel's sign and Phalen's test in carpal tunnel syndrome. Orthopedics 1992;15(11):1297–302.

42. Hartz CR, Linscheid RL, Gramse RR, et al. The pronator teres syndrome: compressive neuropathy of the median nerve. J Bone Joint Surg Am 1981; 63(6):885–90.

43. Gainor BJ. The pronator compression test revisited. A forgotten physical sign. Orthop Rev 1990; 19(10):888–92.

44. Toia F, Gagliardo A, D'Arpa S, et al. Preoperative evaluation of peripheral nerve injuries: what is the place for ultrasound? J Neurosurg 2016;125(3): 603–14.

45. Khachi G, Skirgaudes M, Lee WP, et al. The clinical applications of peripheral nerve imaging in the upper extremity. J Hand Surg Am 2007;32(10): 1600–4.

46. Toros T, Karabay N, Ozaksar K, et al. Evaluation of peripheral nerves of the upper limb with ultrasonography: a comparison of ultrasonographic examination and the intra-operative findings. J Bone Joint Surg Br 2009;91(6):762–5.

47. Cartwright MS, Chloros GD, Walker FO, et al. Diagnostic ultrasound for nerve transection. Muscle Nerve 2007;35(6):796–9.

48. Duetzmann S, Tas S, Seifert V, et al. Cross-sectional area of the median nerve before revision carpal tunnel release-A cross-sectional study. Oper Neurosurg (Hagerstown) 2018;14(1):20–5.

49. Shapiro SA, Alkhamisi A, Pujalte GG. Sonographic appearance of the median nerve following revision

carpal tunnel surgery. J Clin Imaging Sci 2016;6: 11.

50. Watson JC. The electrodiagnostic approach to carpal tunnel syndrome. Neurol Clin 2012;30(2): 457–78.

51. Osiak K, Mazurek A, Pekala P, et al. Electrodiagnostic studies in the surgical treatment of carpal tunnel syndrome-A systematic review. J Clin Med 2021;(12):10.

52. Lo SF, Chou LW, Meng NH, et al. Clinical characteristics and electrodiagnostic features in patients with carpal tunnel syndrome, double crush syndrome, and cervical radiculopathy. Rheumatol Int 2012;32(5):1257–63.

53. Vora AM, Schon LC. Revision peripheral nerve surgery. Foot Ankle Clin 2004;9(2):305–18.

54. Campagna R, Pessis E, Feydy A, et al. MRI assessment of recurrent carpal tunnel syndrome after open surgical release of the median nerve. AJR Am J Roentgenol 2009;193(3):644–50.

55. Taghizadeh R, Tahir A, Stevenson S, et al. The role of MRI in the diagnosis of recurrent/persistent carpal tunnel syndrome: a radiological and intraoperative correlation. J Plast Reconstr Aesthet Surg 2011;64(9):1250–2.

56. Wu HT, Schweitzer ME, Culp RW. Potential MR signs of recurrent carpal tunnel syndrome: initial experience. J Comput Assist Tomogr 2004;28(6):860–4.

57. Beck JD, Brothers JG, Maloney PJ, et al. Predicting the outcome of revision carpal tunnel release. J Hand Surg Am 2012;37(2):282–7.

58. Botte MJ, von Schroeder HP, Abrams RA, et al. Recurrent carpal tunnel syndrome. Hand Clin 1996;12(4):731–43.

59. Gould D, Kulber D, Kuschner S, et al. Our surgical experience: open versus endoscopic carpal tunnel surgery. J Hand Surg Am 2018;43(9):853–61.

60. Luria S, Waitayawinyu T, Trumble TE. Endoscopic revision of carpal tunnel release. Plast Reconstr Surg 2008;121(6):2029–34.

61. Fried SM, Nazarian LN. Ultrasound-guided hydroneurolysis of the median nerve for recurrent carpal tunnel syndrome. Hand (N Y) 2019;14(3):413–21.

62. Langdell HC, Zeng SL, Pidgeon TS, et al. Recalcitrant neuropathies in the upper extremity. J Hand Surg Glob Online 2023;5(4):503–9.

63. Pourmand R, Ochs S, Jersild RA Jr. The relation of the beading of myelinated nerve fibers to the bands of Fontana. Neuroscience 1994;61(2): 373–80.

64. Hunter JM. Recurrent carpal tunnel syndrome, epineural fibrous fixation, and traction neuropathy. Hand Clin 1991;7(3):491–504.

65. Duclos L, Sokolow C. Management of true recurrent carpal tunnel syndrome: is it worthwhile to bring vascularized tissue? Chir Main 1998;17(2): 113–7 [discussion 118].

66. Pizzillo MF, Sotereanos DG, Tomaino MM. Recurrent carpal tunnel syndrome: treatment options. J South Orthop Associng 1999;8(1):28–36.

67. Mackinnon SE, McCabe S, Murray JF, et al. Internal neurolysis fails to improve the results of primary carpal tunnel decompression. J Hand Surg Am 1991;16(2):211–8.

68. Gelberman RH, Pfeffer GB, Galbraith RT, et al. Results of treatment of severe carpal-tunnel syndrome without internal neurolysis of the median nerve. J Bone Joint Surg Am 1987;69(6):896–903.

69. Soltani AM, Allan BJ, Best MJ, et al. A systematic review of the literature on the outcomes of treatment for recurrent and persistent carpal tunnel syndrome. Plast Reconstr Surg 2013;132(1): 114–21.

70. Curtis RM, Eversmann WW Jr. Internal neurolysis as an adjunct to the treatment of the carpal-tunnel syndrome. J Bone Joint Surg Am 1973; 55(4):733–40.

71. Rhoades CE, Mowery CA, Gelberman RH. Results of internal neurolysis of the median nerve for severe carpal-tunnel syndrome. J Bone Joint Surg Am 1985;67(2):253–6.

72. Strickland JW, Idler RS, Lourie GM, et al. The hypothenar fat pad flap for management of recalcitrant carpal tunnel syndrome. J Hand Surg Am 1996;21(5):840–8.

73. Abzug JM, Jacoby SM, Osterman AL. Surgical options for recalcitrant carpal tunnel syndrome with perineural fibrosis. Hand (N Y) 2012;7(1):23–9.

74. Mosier BA, Hughes TB. Recurrent carpal tunnel syndrome. Hand Clin 2013;29(3):427–34.

75. Craft RO, Duncan SF, Smith AA. Management of recurrent carpal tunnel syndrome with microneurolysis and the hypothenar fat pad flap. Hand (N Y) 2007;2(3):85–9.

76. Jansen MC, Duraku LS, Hundepool CA, et al. Management of recurrent carpal tunnel syndrome: systematic review and meta-analysis. J Hand Surg Am 2022;47(4):388 e1–e388. e19.

77. Koncilia H, Kuzbari R, Worseg A, et al. The lumbrical muscle flap: anatomic study and clinical application. J Hand Surg Am 1998;23(1):111–9.

78. Milward TM, Stott WG, Kleinert HE. The abductor digiti minimi muscle flap. Hand 1977;9(1):82–5.

79. Dellon AL, Mackinnon SE. The pronator quadratus muscle flap. J Hand Surg Am 1984;9(3):423–7.

80. Rose EH, Norris MS, Kowalski TA, et al. Palmaris brevis turnover flap as an adjunct to internal neurolysis of the chronically scarred median nerve in recurrent carpal tunnel syndrome. J Hand Surg Am 1991;16(2):191–201.

81. Tham SK, Ireland DC, Riccio M, et al. Reverse radial artery fascial flap: a treatment for the chronically scarred median nerve in recurrent carpal tunnel syndrome. J Hand Surg Am 1996;21(5):849–54.

82. Murthy PG, Abzug JM, Jacoby SM, et al. The teno-synovial flap for recalcitrant carpal tunnel syndrome. Tech Hand Up Extrem Surg 2013;17(2): 84–6.

83. Goitz RJ, Steichen JB. Microvascular omental transfer for the treatment of severe recurrent median neuritis of the wrist: a long-term follow-up. Plast Reconstr Surg 2005;115(1):163–71.

84. Dahlin LB, Lekholm C, Kardum P, et al. Coverage of the median nerve with free and pedicled flaps for the treatment of recurrent severe carpal tunnel syndrome. Scand J Plast ReConstr Surg Hand Surg 2002;36(3):172–6.

85. Wintsch K, Helaly P. Free flap of gliding tissue. J Reconstr Microsurg 1986;2(3):143–51.

86. Dy CJ, Aunins B, Brogan DM. Barriers to epineural Scarring: role in treatment of traumatic nerve injury and chronic compressive neuropathy. J Hand Surg Am 2018;43(4):360–7.

87. Goldfarb CA, Sutter MM, Martens EJ, et al. Incidence of re-operation and subjective outcome following in situ decompression of the ulnar nerve at the cubital tunnel. J Hand Surg Eur 2009;34(3): 379–83.

88. Gaspar MP, Kane PM, Putthiwara D, et al. Predicting revision following in situ ulnar nerve decompression for patients with idiopathic cubital tunnel syndrome. J Hand Surg Am 2016;41(3):427–35.

89. Krogue JD, Aleem AW, Osei DA, et al. Predictors of surgical revision after in situ decompression of the ulnar nerve. J Shoulder Elbow Surg 2015;24(4): 634–9.

90. Amadio PC. Anatomical basis for a technique of ulnar nerve transposition. Surg Radiol Anat 1986; 8(3):155–61.

91. Burahee AS, Sanders AD, Power DM. The management of failed cubital tunnel decompression. EFORT Open Rev 2021;6(9):735–42.

92. Nellans K, Tang P. Evaluation and treatment of failed ulnar nerve release at the elbow. Orthop Clin North Am 2012;43(4):487–94.

93. Davidge KM, Ebersole GC, Mackinnon SE. Pain and function following revision cubital tunnel surgery. Hand (N Y) 2019;14(2):172–8.

94. Mackinnon SE, Novak CB. Operative findings in re-operation of patients with cubital tunnel syndrome. Hand (N Y) 2007;2(3):137–43.

95. Spinner M, Kaplan EB. The relationship of the ulnar nerve to the medial intermuscular septum in the arm and its clinical significance. Hand 1976;8(3): 239–42.

96. Dellon AL, MacKinnon SE. Injury to the medial antebrachial cutaneous nerve during cubital tunnel surgery. J Hand Surg Br 1985;10(1):33–6.

97. Tanaka SK, Lourie GM. Anatomic course of the medial antebrachial cutaneous nerve: a cadaveric study with proposed clinical application in failed

cubital tunnel release. J Hand Surg Eur Vol 2015; 40(2):210–2.

98. Aleem AW, Krogue JD, Calfee RP. Outcomes of revision surgery for cubital tunnel syndrome. J Hand Surg Am 2014;39(11):2141–9.

99. Smit JA, Hu Y, Brohet RM, et al. Identifying risk factors for recurrence after cubital tunnel release. J Hand Surg Am 2023;48(5):514 e1–e514 e7.

100. Spinner RJ, Goldner RD. Snapping of the medial head of the triceps and recurrent dislocation of the ulnar nerve. Anatomical and dynamic factors. J Bone Joint Surg Am 1998;80(2):239–47.

101. Davidge KM, Gontre G, Tang D, et al. The "hierarchical" Scratch Collapse Test for identifying multi-level ulnar nerve compression. Hand (N Y) 2015; 10(3):388–95.

102. Lauder A, Chen C, Bolson RM, et al. Management of recalcitrant cubital tunnel syndrome. J Am Acad Orthop Surg 2021;29(15):635–47.

103. Boers N, Brakkee EM, Krijgh DD, et al. The diagnostic role of ultrasound in cubital tunnel syndrome for patients with a previous cubital tunnel surgery. J Plast Reconstr Aesthet Surg 2022;75(11):4063–8.

104. Dagregorio G, Saint-Cast Y. Simple neurolysis for failed anterior submuscular transposition of the ulnar nerve at the elbow. Int Orthop 2004;28(6): 342–6.

105. Jaddue DA, Saloo SA, Sayed-Noor AS. Subcutaneous vs submuscular ulnar nerve transposition in Moderate cubital tunnel syndrome. Open Orthop J 2009;3:78–82.

106. Staples JR, Calfee R. Cubital tunnel syndrome: current concepts. J Am Acad Orthop Surg 2017; 25(10):e215–24.

107. Wever N, de Ruiter GCW, Coert JH. Submuscular transposition with musculofascial lengthening for persistent or recurrent cubital tunnel syndrome in 34 patients. J Hand Surg Eur Vol 2018;43(3):310–5.

108. Caputo AE, Watson HK. Subcutaneous anterior transposition of the ulnar nerve for failed decompression of cubital tunnel syndrome. J Hand Surg Am 2000;25(3):544–51.

109. Charles YP, Coulet B, Rouzaud JC, et al. Comparative clinical outcomes of submuscular and subcutaneous transposition of the ulnar nerve for cubital tunnel syndrome. J Hand Surg Am May-Jun 2009;34(5):866–74.

110. Richmond JC, Southmayd WW. Superficial anterior transposition of the ulnar nerve at the elbow for ulnar neuritis. Clin Orthop Relat Res 1982;(164): 42 4.

111. Danoff JR, Lombardi JM, Rosenwasser MP. Use of a pedicled adipose flap as a sling for anterior subcutaneous transposition of the ulnar nerve. J Hand Surg Am 2014;39(3):552–5.

112. Verveld CJ, Danoff JR, Lombardi JM, et al. Adipose flap versus fascial sling for anterior subcutaneous

transposition of the ulnar nerve. Am J Orthop (Belle Mead NJ) 2016;45(2):89–94.

113. Gaspar MP, Abdelfattah HM, Welch IW, et al. Recurrent cubital tunnel syndrome treated with revision neurolysis and amniotic membrane nerve wrapping. J Shoulder Elbow Surg 2016;25(12):2057–65.

114. Kokkalis ZT, Jain S, Sotereanos DG. Vein wrapping at cubital tunnel for ulnar nerve problems. J Shoulder Elbow Surg 2010;19(2 Suppl):91–7.

115. Papatheodorou LK, Williams BG, Sotereanos DG. Preliminary results of recurrent cubital tunnel syndrome treated with neurolysis and porcine extracellular matrix nerve wrap. J Hand Surg Am 2015;40(5):987–92.

116. Barbour J, Yee A, Kahn LC, et al. Supercharged end-to-side anterior interosseous to ulnar motor nerve transfer for intrinsic musculature reinnervation. J Hand Surg Am 2012;37(10):2150–9.

117. Dengler J, Dolen U, Patterson JMM, et al. Supercharge end-to-side anterior interosseous-to-ulnar motor nerve transfer restores intrinsic function in cubital tunnel syndrome. Plast Reconstr Surg 2020;146(4):808–18.

118. Doherty CD, Miller TA, Larocerie-Salgado J, et al. Reverse end-to-side anterior interosseous nerve-to-ulnar motor transfer for severe ulnar neuropathy. Plast Reconstr Surg 2020;146(3):306e–13e.

119. Head LK, Zhang ZZ, Hicks K, et al. Evaluation of intrinsic hand musculature reinnervation following Supercharge end-to-side anterior interosseous-to-ulnar motor nerve transfer. Plast Reconstr Surg 2020;146(1):128–32.

120. Baltzer H, Woo A, Oh C, et al. Comparison of ulnar intrinsic function following supercharge end-to-side anterior interosseous-to-ulnar motor nerve transfer: a matched cohort study of proximal ulnar nerve injury patients. Plast Reconstr Surg 2016;138(6):1264–72.

121. Power HA, Kahn LC, Patterson MM, et al. Refining indications for the supercharge end-to-side anterior interosseous to ulnar motor nerve transfer in cubital tunnel syndrome. Plast Reconstr Surg 2020;145(1):106e–16e.

Nerve Versus Tendon Transfers in the Management of Isolated Upper Extremity Peripheral Nerve Injuries

Dexter W. Weeks, MD[a], Ronald D. Brown, MD[b],*

KEYWORDS

- Peripheral nerve injury • Upper extremity nerve injury • Nerve transfers in upper extremity
- Tendon transfers in upper extremity

KEY POINTS

- Upper extremity peripheral nerve injuries may be treated by tendon or nerve transfers.
- Tendon transfers require supple joints, adequate soft tissue envelope, expendable and synergistic donor tendons, and maximally straight vector of pull.
- Nerve transfers are used when long reinnervation distance is expected, the recipient is close to the donor nerve, and the donor and recipient are synergistic.
- Tendon transfers should have optimal tension to maximize postoperative functional outcomes.
- Nerve transfers should be performed without undue tension at the coaptation site and with adequate soft tissue coverage.

INTRODUCTION

Approximately 3% of patients treated in level 1 trauma centers suffer from peripheral nerve injury.[1,2] Sixty percent of patients with these injuries present during emergent or urgent admissions.[3] Tendon transfers date to the nineteenth century, with application in paralytic sequelae of polio infection.[4–6] The widespread application of tendon transfer principles bloomed in the twentieth century, following the World Wars.[6–10] Nerve transfers developed similarly, with early use for war-time injuries, and more widespread applications in upper extremity injuries later.[11–15] More robust comprehension of upper extremity peripheral nerve injury[16,17] proliferated tendon and nerve transfer techniques. Despite the lack of consensus regarding optimal surgical procedure,[18–20,22] the expansile nature of these tools offer great potential for satisfactory outcomes.

PRINCIPLES OF TENDON TRANSFER

Essential principles of tendon transfer include supple joints at the site of desired motion, adequate soft tissue envelope, and expendable, synergistic donor tendons of adequate excursion and strength with a straight vector of pull.[6,21,23,24,25,26,28,31] Expected tendon excursion is 3 cm for wrist flexors and extensors, 5 cm for extrinsic digital extensors, and 7 cm for extrinsic digital flexors.[4,10,27] The donor muscle–tendon

a Department of Orthopaedic Surgery, The Ohio State University Hand and Upper Extremity Center, 915 Olentangy River Road, Suite 3200, Columbus, OH 43210, USA; b Hand and Plastic Surgery, Department of Plastic and Reconstructive Surgery, The Ohio State University Hand and Upper Extremity Center, 915 Olentangy River Road, Suite 3200, Columbus, OH 43212, USA
* Corresponding author.
E-mail address: Ronald.Brown@osumc.edu

Clin Plastic Surg 51 (2024) 473–483
https://doi.org/10.1016/j.cps.2024.02.013
0094-1298/24/© 2024 Elsevier Inc. All rights reserved.

unit (MTU) should be normal or near-normal in strength, as the donor muscle will lose one functional grade with transfer.[6,21,28]

PRINCIPLES OF NERVE TRANSFER

Nerve transfers can lead to earlier muscle reinnervation, restore sensation, and avoid additional surgery in scarred beds. Synergism is prioritized as it simplifies re-education.[28] The surgeon should consider nerve transfers when the reinnervation distance is long, the desired target is in proximity to the donor nerve, and the donor is synergistic to the recipient.[2,29] Nerve coaptations are performed in tension-free end-to-end manner.[30] Optimal timing is 4 to 6 months after injury to avoid the irreversible motor endplate loss that occurs around 1 year. Reinnervation of injured muscle does not alter its biomechanical structure, excursion, attachments, or length–tension relationships. Minimal immobilization is required, facilitating early active motion.[29]

Low Radial Nerve Palsy Tendon Transfers

Functional goals of tendon transfers for low radial nerve palsy include digital metacarpophalangeal joint (MPJ) and thumb interphalangeal joint (IPJ) extension. Notably, the proximally innervated extensor carpi radialis longus (ECRL) remains intact (innervated by radial nerve proper) in "low" radial nerve injuries.

Restoring finger extension in radial nerve palsy is well described as flexor carpi radialis (FCR) to extensor digitorum communis (EDC) transfer.[4,6,28,31] Advocates for FCR donor, as opposed to flexor carpi ulnaris (FCU), endorse ease of dissection and maintaining ulnar deviation at the wrist.[6,28]

Thumb IPJ extension can be restored via palmaris longus (PL) to extensor pollicis longus (EPL) or flexor digitorum superficialis (FDS) of ring to EPL transfers.[6,28,31] The authors' preferred transfers for low radial nerve palsy include FCR to EDC and PL to EPL.

Flexor carpi radialis to extensor digitorum communis transfer

The FCR is divided at the distal wrist crease and routed subcutaneously along the radial border of the forearm or through the interosseous membrane. The EDC tendons are divided distal to the musculotendinous junction and sutured together. The distal FCR tendon end is attached end-to-side to the EDC tendon mass proximal to the extensor retinaculum (**Fig. 1**). Tensioning of the transfer is set with the wrist in slight extension and the MPJs in full extension.

Palmaris longus to extensor palmaris longus transfer

The PL tendon is identified and divided at the distal wrist crease and routed subcutaneously around the radial forearm. The EPL tendon is divided at its musculotendinous junction and retracted distally out of the third extensor compartment to create a straight vector of pull. The PL tendon is then sutured to the EPL tendon in a Pulvertaft weave. Tensioning is performed with the thumb in maximal extension at the MPJ and IPJ.

Low Radial Nerve Palsy Nerve Transfers

Branches of the median nerve are optimal donors for low radial nerve palsy.[32–34,36,37] The synergism of wrist flexion with digital and wrist extension with digital flexion capitalizes on tenodesis to produce gripping. The preferred nerve transfers for low radial nerve palsy are FDS branch to extensor carpi radialis brevis (ECRB) to restore wrist extension and FCR branch to posterior interosseous nerve (PIN).[32–35] These transfers should be performed in tandem and not isolation. An alternative is the AIN to ECRB motor branch and nerve to FCR to PIN transfers **Fig. 2**, as described by Bertelli.[31]

Technique

The superficial sensory branch of the radial nerve (SBRN) is identified beneath the brachioradialis (BR) and followed proximally until PIN and trunk of the radial nerve are identified. The PIN branch to the ECRB is exposed by dividing the tendinous origin of the ECRB as well as the leash of Henry. The PIN branch to ECRB runs parallel and radial to SBRN. The PIN proper will be identified deep to supinator muscle. The arcade of Frohse can be released to allow more mobilization of the PIN.

The median nerve is then identified in the distal forearm and followed proximally until it courses between the heads of pronator teres (PT). The heads of PT should be elevated from the median nerve to allow decompression and easier identification of the target branches. The branches to FDS are exposed by releasing the FDS arch. The branches will be taking off from the ulnar aspect of the median nerve and into the FDS muscle belly. More proximal dissection will reveal the FCR motor branch. Hand-held nerve stimulator can aid in identification.

The FCR and FDS branches are divided distally at the muscle bellies and transposed radially toward their respective targets. The recipient PIN and ECRB branches are divided proximally and transposed ulnarly toward the donor nerves to facilitate tension-free coaptation. Coaptations are

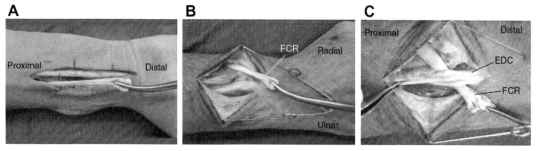

Fig. 1. A cadaver demonstrating the flexor carpi radialis (FCR) to extensor digitorum communis (EDC) tendon transfer for restoration of finger extension. (*A*) A radial incision is made over the FCR tendon for harvest. The FCR tendon is divided starting at the wrist crease (*B*), routed dorsoradially around the forearm (*C*), and attached end-to-side and en mass to each of the EDC tendons. (*From* Seiler JG 3rd, Desai MJ, Payne SH. Tendon transfers for radial, median, and ulnar nerve palsy. J Am Acad Orthop Surg. 2013 Nov;21(11):675-84. PMID 24187037.)

performed under microscopy with 9-0 nylon suture.

High Radial Nerve Palsy Tendon Transfers

High radial nerve palsy includes an inability to extend the wrist. Wrist extension is accomplished using a PT to ECRB transfer. Finger and thumb extension is addressed as described for low radial nerve palsy (**Table 1**).

Pronator teres to extensor carpi radialis brevis tendon transfer

A longitudinal incision is made over the volar and radial mid-forearm. The PT can be identified deep to BR, in an interval between SBRN and radial artery. The PT insertion onto the radius is elevated with a strip of periosteum to increase length. The tendon is dissected proximally toward its musculotendinous junction, freeing any surrounding soft tissue attachments.

The ECRL and ECRB tendons are identified through a separate dorsal wrist incision. The ECRB tendon is divided at its musculotendinous

junction. The mobilized PT tendon is routed subcutaneously around the radial forearm, superficial to BR and ECRL, and sutured end-to-end with the distal ECRB tendon. Tensioning is done with wrist extended to 45°.

High Radial Nerve Palsy Nerve Transfers

Nerve transfers for high radial nerve palsy remain the same as those for low palsy and are listed in **Table 2**.

Low Median Nerve Palsy Tendon Transfers

Thumb opposition is absent in low median nerve palsy. Restoration of thumb opposition relies on donor attachment to the abductor pollicis brevis (APB).[38–42,43,51] The extensor indicis proprius (EIP) to APB opponensplasty can be applied in high and low median nerve palsies,[44,47] whereas PL to APB is frequently performed in severe carpal tunnel syndrome.[51] There are no strong data to show functional superiority between opponensplasty techniques.[51] The authors' preferred techniques include PL to APB and EIP to APB.

Fig. 2. Intraoperative view of AIN to ECRB motor branch and nerve to FCR to PIN transfers. (*From* Bertelli JA. Nerve versus tendon transfer for radial nerve paralysis reconstruction. J Hand Surg Am. 2020 May;45(5):418-426. PMID 32093993.)

Table 1	
Tendon transfers in radial nerve palsy	
Functional Deficit	**Tendon Transfer Options**
Thumb Extension	PL to EPL
	FDS (ring) to EPL
Digital Extension	FCR to EDC
	FDS to EDC
	FCU to EDC
Wrist Extension	PT to ECRB

Abbreviations: ECRB, extensor carpi radialis brevis; EDC, extensor digitorum communis; EPL, extensor pollicis longus; FCR, flexor carpi radialis; FCU, flexor carpi ulnaris; FDS, flexor digitorum superficialis; PL, palmaris longus; PT, pronator teres.

Table 2		
Nerve transfers in radial nerve palsy		
Functional Deficit	Donor Nerve	Recipient Nerve
Wrist and digital extension	Median nerve branch to FDS	Radial nerve branch to ECRB
	Median nerve branch to FCR	PIN

Abbreviations: ECRB, extensor carpi radialis brevis; FCR, flexor carpi radialis; FDS, flexor digitorum superficialis; PIN, posterior interosseous nerve.

Palmaris longus to abductor pollicis brevis transfer

A longitudinal incision in line with the ring finger ray is made over the volar forearm and proximal palm. The PL is identified and freed from palm to the musculotendinous junction in the forearm along with a 1–2 cm-wide strip of the palmar aponeurosis. This fascial extension serves to lengthen the PL for transfer. The APB insertion is exposed at the thumb MPJ (metacarpophalangeal joint) via a second incision. The PL tendon strip is tunneled subcutaneously and delivered to the dorsoradial thumb incision and sutured to the APB insertion and dorsal MPJ capsule. Tension is set with the wrist in neutral posture, the thumb MPJ in extension, and the thumb in full opposition.

Extensor indicis proprius to abductor pollicis brevis transfer

The EIP to APB transfer is depicted in **Fig. 3**. The EIP tendon is identified at the dorsal MP and divided just proximal to its coalition with the extensor hood. A second incision is made at the dorsal wrist and the EIP tendon is retracted proximally through the fourth extensor compartment, proximal to the extensor retinaculum. A third incision is made at the dorsoradial thumb MP joint exposing the APB insertion and a fourth incision is made on the volar ulnar wrist, proximal to the pisiform. The EIP tendon is then tunneled subcutaneously around the ulnar forearm to the volar ulnar wrist incision, after which it is tunneled subcutaneously to the radial thumb incision. The EIP tendon is then sutured to the APB insertion. Tensioning is performed with the wrist in neutral and thumb in maximum opposition.

Low Median Nerve Palsy Nerve Transfers

Limited literature has been published on nerve transfers in low median nerve injuries. Mackinnon and colleagues described an anterior interosseous nerve (AIN) branch to pronator quadratus (PQ) to median recurrent motor branch for thumb opposition.[29,30]

One caveat of this technique is it may require an interposition nerve graft for adequate length.

Anterior interosseous nerve (pronator quadratus) to recurrent median motor branch transfer

A carpal tunnel incision is made on the volar palm, extending 4 cm proximal to the distal wrist crease. The median nerve is identified and dissected distally until the recurrent motor branch is identified. The recurrent motor branch is transected proximally at its branching point. Attention is then turned to the proximal aspect of the incision where the PQ muscle can be identified. The AIN branch is visualized entering the deep and proximal aspect of PQ. A longitudinal myotomy of PQ is performed to visualize the most distal extent of the AIN and it is transected prior to its arborization within the muscle. A harvested nerve graft is then coapted to the distal aspect of the AIN, delivered along the course of the median nerve, and finally coapted distally to the cut end of the recurrent median motor branch.

High Median Nerve Palsy Tendon Transfers

Flexion in the index and long fingers are restored using an ECRL to flexor digitorum profundus (FDP) transfer.[23] The ECRL donor is optimal because it allows independent flexion of the digits as opposed to the obligate composite flexion in a side-to-side FDP tenodesis. Radially innervated BR can be used to restore thumb IPJ flexion[23] (**Table 3**).

Extensor carpi radialis longus to flexor digitorum profundus transfer

The ECRL is identified and detached from the second metacarpal base via a dorsal incision. The FDP tendons are identified through a separate volar Henry incision. The FDP to index and long fingers are divided transversely at the musculotendinous junction. The ECRL tendon is routed subcutaneously along the radial forearm, deep to the BR tendon. The ECRL is then sutured to the index and long finger FDP tendons in end-to-end manner. The transfer is tensioned with the wrist extended to 30° and the digits in full flexion; wrist flexion to 30° should create full extension of the index and long fingers.

Brachioradialis to flexor pollicis longus transfer

The BR is identified and detached from the radial styloid via a modified Henry approach. The interval between the FCR and BR is developed to expose the flexor pollicis longus (FPL) muscle which can then be divided at its musculotendinous junction. The distal BR tendon is transferred

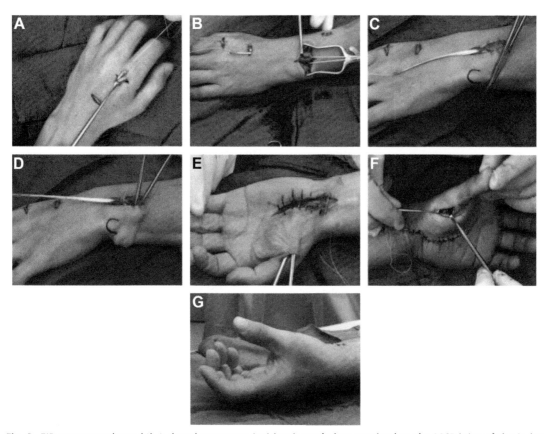

Fig. 3. EIP opponensplasty. (*A*) A dorsal transverse incision is made just proximal to the MCP joint of the index finger, and the EIP is transected proximal to the sagittal bands. (*B, C*) Identification of the EIP musculotendinous junction through an incision made over fourth extensor compartment. Fascial attachments are divided and the EIP is pulled proximally into this incision. (*D*) A subcutaneous tunnel is developed around the ulna and (*E*) also between the pisiform and the insertion site over the radial border of the thumb MCP. In the setting of a concurrent carpal tunnel release, as in this patient, an extensile carpal tunnel incision replaces the need for an incision just proximal to the pisiform. The EIP is passed subcutaneously around the ulna, into the carpal tunnel incision, then to the incision at the radial border of the thumb. (*F*) The tendon is sutured into place. (*G*) Appropriate tensioning results in the thumb resting palmarly abducted and opposite the index and middle fingers with the wrist at neutral. (*From* Chadderdon RC, Gaston RG. Low median nerve transfers (opponensplasty). Hand Clin. 2016 Aug;32(3):349-59. PMID: 27387078.)

Table 3
Tendon transfers in median nerve palsy

Functional Deficit	Tendon Transfer Options
Thumb Opposition	PL to APB
	FDS (ring) to APB
	ADM to APB
	EIP to APB
Digital Flexion	ECRL to FDP
	FDP side-to-side tenodesis
Thumb Flexion	BR to FPL

Abbreviations: ADM, abductor digiti minimi; APB, abductor pollicis brevis; BR, brachioradialis; ECRL, extensor carpi radialis longus; EIP, extensor indicis proprius; FDP, flexor digitorum profundus; FDS, flexor digitorum superficialis; FPL, flexor pollicis longus; PL, palmaris longus.

to the FPL tendon, and tension is set with the wrist at neutral and the thumb MPJ and IPJ in 30° flexion.

High Median Nerve Palsy Nerve Transfers

Restoration of wrist and digital flexion, as well as pronation, is necessary in high median nerve palsy. The recommended transfers are ECRB to AIN transfer and motor branch of supinator to PT32 (**Table 4**).

Surgical technique

A longitudinal curvilinear incision is made on the volar forearm and the SBRN is identified beneath the BR tendon and dissected proximally to its

Table 4
Nerve transfers in median nerve palsy

Nerve Injury	Functional Deficit	Donor Nerve	Recipient Nerve
Low Median Nerve Palsy	Thumb opposition	AIN (PQ)	Median recurrent motor branch
High Median Nerve Palsy	Thumb opposition, wrist and digital flexion, forearm pronation	Radial nerve branch to ECRB	AIN
		Radial nerve branch to supinator	Median motor branch to PT

Abbreviations: AIN, anterior interosseous nerve; ECRB, extensor carpi radialis brevis; PQ, pronator quadratus; PT, pronator teres.

branch point from the radial nerve. The PIN branch to the ECRB runs parallel and radial to SBRN and is exposed by dividing the tendinous origin of the ECRB and the leash of Henry.

The median nerve is then identified in the distal forearm and followed proximally until it courses between the heads of PT. The heads of PT should be elevated from the median nerve to allow decompression. The AIN will be identified as it arises from the radial side of the main median nerve trunk.

The PIN branch to ECRB is divided at its interface with the muscle and neurolysed from the arcade of Frohse to allow mobilization ulnarly. The AIN is then transected at its origin from the median nerve and coapted to the PIN branch to ECRB in an end-to-end manner.

Next, the PIN branch to supinator is identified on the muscle's deep surface and divided. Branches from the median nerve going to the deep aspect of PT are identified and followed proximally toward the antecubital fossa where they are transected distal to their origin. The distal aspect of the PIN branch to supinator is then transposed and coapted end-to-end with the proximal aspect of the median nerve branch to PT.

Low Ulnar Nerve Palsy Tendon Transfers

Claw deformity correction is imperative for effective grip strength.[51,52] Dynamic procedures transfer the FDS or ECRB tendons. The preferred FDS transfers are the Zancolli lasso[51] (**Fig. 4**) and modified Stiles–Bunnell transfers.[52] The advantage of the Zancolli lasso is simplicity when compared to modified Stiles–Bunnell. In contrast, the modified Stiles–Bunnell may achieve greater flexion synchrony compared to the Zancolli procedure.[23,45,46,48,49,50,51,52]

The ECRB transfer described by Brand also corrects claw deformity.[53] However, criticisms of the technique include difficulty in patient re-education and the need for interposition tendon grafts.[52]

Surgical restoration of key pinch is accomplished by ECRB to adductor pollicis (AP) transfer with free tendon interposition graft. Alternatively, FDS of ring or long finger to AP transfer may be performed (**Table 5**). The authors' preferred technique is the modified Stiles–Bunnell.

Modified Stiles–Bunnell transfer

A volar Bruner incision is made over the PIPJ (proximal interphalangeal joint) of the middle or

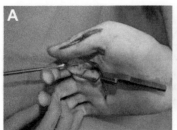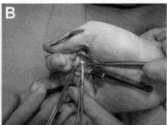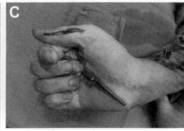

Fig. 4. Zancolli lasso procedure. (*A*) Flexor tendon sheath (*) identified and a window is made in the distal A2 pulley (). (*B*) FDS tendon (+) transected distally at its insertion. (*C*) FDS tendon (+) looped proximally over the A1 pulley (–) and sutured on itself. (*From* Starr BW, Chung KC. Dynamic rather than static procedures in correcting claw deformities due to ulnar nerve palsy. Hand Clin. 2022 Aug; 38(3):313-319. PMID 35985755.)

Table 5
Tendon transfers in ulnar nerve palsy

Functional Deficit	Tendon Transfer Options
Clawing	FDS (Zancolli) lasso FDS (modified Stiles–Bunnell) ECRB (Brand)
Thumb Adduction	ECRB to AP FDS to AP
Ring and Small Finger DIPJ Flexion	FDP side-to-side tenodesis

Abbreviations: AP, adductor pollicis; ECRB, extensor carpi radialis brevis; FDP, flexor digitorum profundus; FDS, flexor digitorum superficialis.

Table 6
Nerve transfers in ulnar nerve palsy

Functional Deficit	Donor Nerve	Recipient Nerve
Clawing, intrinsic weakness, loss of thumb adduction, loss of ring, and small finger DIPJ flexion	Distal AIN	Ulnar motor branch

Abbreviation: AIN, anterior interosseous nerve.

ring finger, and subcutaneous dissection proceeds to the flexor tendon sheath. The flexor sheath is incised and both slips of FDS are transected proximal to Camper chiasm while FDP is protected.

A second transverse incision is made at the distal palmar crease, and proximally directed traction is applied to the previously transected FDS tendons to retract the tendon ends to the palmar incision. Both slips of FDS are longitudinally divided as far proximally as visible to create 4 separate tendon slips.

Next, midaxial incisions are made along the radial aspect of the ring and small finger PIPJs and the lateral bands are exposed. Subcutaneous tunnels are created from the midaxial incisions, proximally through the lumbrical canals, and to the FDS donor tendons located in the palm. The tunnel should be volar to the deep transverse metacarpal ligaments. The FDS tendon slips are delivered distally through these tunnels to the lateral bands.

A longitudinal incision is made in the midline of the radial lateral band. The FDS tendon slip is woven through the radial lateral band incision and woven onto itself. Tension is set with the wrist at neutral and the MPJs at 60° flexion.

Low Ulnar Nerve Palsy Nerve Transfers

Distal AIN to ulnar nerve deep motor branch (UMN) transfer is recommended for ulnar nerve palsy.[11,32,53] This transfer offers the potential to obviate tendon transfers in ulnar nerve palsy (**Table 6**).

Distal anterior interosseous nerve to ulnar motor nerve branch transfer

A curvilinear ulnar palm incision is designed with Bruner extension across the distal wrist crease and terminating in the distal ulnar forearm (**Fig. 5**). Subcutaneous dissection in the distal forearm and palm is performed until the ulnar nerve is identified in Guyon canal. Gentle traction is applied to the ulnar neurovascular bundle to reveal the deep motor branch of ulnar nerve running ulnar to the hook of the hamate and deep to the hypothenar musculature (**Fig. 6**). The proximal fascial edge of the hypothenar muscles is longitudinally divided to completely decompress the deep motor branch.[32,53]

The motor branch of the ulnar nerve is traced proximally into the forearm and can be internally neurolysed proximally to ensure isolation of the motor fibers. A vessel loop can be placed around the motor fascicular group to isolate it in preparation for nerve coaptation (**Fig. 7**). Topographically, the motor branch should lie sandwiched between the 2 sensory branches.

Next, the interval between FCU and PL is developed to expose PQ muscle. Inspection of the proximal edge of PQ will reveal the AIN entering the deep surface of PQ. The PQ is longitudinally divided to expose the distal arborization of the AIN where it can be transected and transposed ulnarly (**Fig. 8**). The AIN can then be transposed

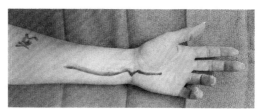

Fig. 5. AIN to UMN transfer. The skin incision is depicted ulnar to the thenar crease, extended across the wrist in a Bruner manner, and extended to the midforearm. (*From* Peters BR, Van Handel AC, Russo SA, Moore AM. Five reliable nerve transfers for the treatment of isolated upper extremity nerve injuries. Plast Reconstr Surg. 2021 May 1;147(5):830e-845e. PMID 33890905.)

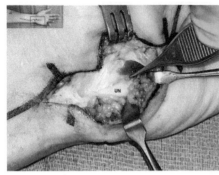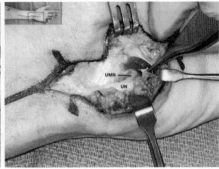

Fig. 6. (*Left*) The proximal, leading edge of the hypothenar fascia (shown at the tip of the forceps) is carefully released to (*right*) decompress the deep motor branch (UMN) of the ulnar nerve (UN). (*From* Peters BR, Van Handel AC, Russo SA, Moore AM. Five reliable nerve transfers for the treatment of isolated upper extremity nerve injuries. Plast Reconstr Surg. 2021 May 1;147(5):830e-845e. PMID 33890905.)

to a site along the ulnar nerve motor branch in a tension-free fashion. This point along the motor nerve is sharply transected and transposed under the flexor tendons toward the AIN where the two can be coapted using the operating microscope (**Fig. 9**). Alternatively, the AIN can be coapted to the ulnar motor branch in end to side fashion if motor recovery is expected.

Postoperative Therapy for Tendon Transfers

The patient is placed in a splint with the elbow flexed to 90° and the wrist in 30° of extension. The joints are positioned to offload the tendon transfers. When appropriate, the IPJs are kept free to range. The postoperative splint is taken down at 2 weeks postoperatively to inspect the incisions and exchange for a thermoplastic splint.

During the first 4 weeks postoperatively, the splint is worn continuously, and the patient is encouraged to range the IPJs of the digits. Between weeks 4 and 6, passive joint mobilization begins, keeping motion limited to a single joint at a time to keep tension off the transfer. At 6 weeks postoperatively, the patient will work with the hand therapist to begin active range of motion exercises. At 8 weeks postoperatively, the patient will wean splint wearing and commence strengthening exercises. Notably, postoperative therapy can vary based on preference and surgical technique.

Postoperative Therapy for Nerve Transfers

The patient is placed in a bulky dressing postoperatively designed to protect the nerve transfer sites. The patient keeps the operated extremity elevated to minimize pain and edema. At 2 to 3 days

Fig. 7. The motor portion of the ulnar nerve (UMN) lies in its ulnar aspect just after the dorsal cutaneous branch (DCU) takeoff in the forearm. It is approximately one-third of the ulnar nerve at this level, and the remaining two-thirds are composed of sensory fascicles (USN). The proximal portion of the pronator quadratus (PQ) has been divided until the anterior interosseous nerve (AIN) begins to branch. (*From* Peters BR, Van Handel AC, Russo SA, Moore AM. Five reliable nerve transfers for the treatment of isolated upper extremity nerve injuries. Plast Reconstr Surg. 2021 May 1;147(5):830e-845e. PMID 33890905.)

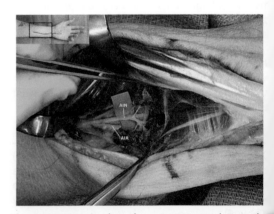

Fig. 8. Just proximal to the pronator quadratus, the anterior interosseous nerve (AIN) runs just radial to the anterior interosseous artery (AIA). (*From* Peters BR, Van Handel AC, Russo SA, Moore AM. Five reliable nerve transfers for the treatment of isolated upper extremity nerve injuries. Plast Reconstr Surg. 2021 Ma 1;147(5):830e-845e. PMID 33890905.)

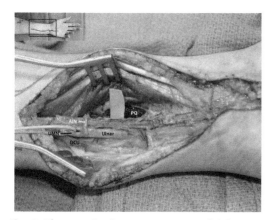

Fig. 9. The anterior interosseous nerve (AIN) supercharge end-to-side coaptation is performed by means of an epineurial and perineurial window in the motor component (UMN) of the ulnar nerve. The pronator quadratus (PQ) and dorsal cutaneous branch (DCU) of the ulnar nerve are also visualized. (*From* Peters BR, Van Handel AC, Russo SA, Moore AM. Five reliable nerve transfers for the treatment of isolated upper extremity nerve injuries. Plast Reconstr Surg. 2021 May 1;147(5):830e-845e. PMID 33890905.)

postoperatively, the dressing is taken down to inspect incisions. A thermoplastic splint for protection and nighttime use is fabricated and used for 3 weeks. The muscle targeted for reinnervation begins resisted exercises to maximize strength. Scar massage is initiated at 1 month postoperatively. Between 8 and 12 weeks postoperatively, strengthening exercises begin. Between 2 and 3 months postoperatively, a nerve study is used to assess early reinnervation.

COMPLICATIONS IN TENDON AND NERVE TRANSFERS

Tendon transfers sacrifice donor muscle function and can result in scarring and adhesions, restricted muscle glide, and decreased strength of transferred tendons. Rupture and adhesion of transferred tendons are possible in inflamed or unstable wound beds with inadequate soft tissue envelope. Often, there is delay in maximal excursion that is improved with postoperative rehabilitation. Tendon rupture or transfer failure can occur and can result from inadequate tendon weaving, premature maximal active range of motion postoperatively, or undue tension on the transfer. In cases where the MTU appears inadequately powered, consider technical factors, such as poor donor selection or improper tensioning of the transfer. Delayed participation in therapy contributes to longer-than-expected functional gains. The surgeon should weight the risks and benefits of

reoperation in relation to expected functional gains of the patient.[21]

Regarding nerve transfers, time to recipient muscle reinnervation is expected to be prolonged, but the surgeon should monitor clinical and functional recovery to optimize transfer timing and donors. Reasons for delayed reinnervation include tension at the coaptation site, infection, or improper nerve selection. Improper nerve selection is avoided by intraoperative nerve stimulation to confirm desired donors and recipients.

SUMMARY

Radial, median, and ulnar nerve injuries present functional deficits that can be managed by both tendon and nerve transfers. To successfully utilize either, the knowledgeable surgeon should be familiar with the principles of tendon and nerve transfers.

CLINICS CARE POINTS

- Recommended tendon transfers in radial nerve palsy include FCR to EDC for digital extension, PL to EPL for thumb extension, and PT to ECRB for wrist extension.

- Recommended nerve transfers include FDS branch to ECRB to restore wrist extension and FCR branch to PIN.

- Recommended tendon transfers in median nerve palsies include PL or EIP to APB for opposition, ECRL to FDP for digital flexion, and BR to FPL for thumb IPJ flexion.

- Recommended nerve transfers in median nerve palsy include motor branch to ECRB to AIN transfer and motor branch of supinator to PT.

- Recommended tendon transfers in ulnar nerve palsy include the modified Stiles-Bunnell transfer or Zancolli lasso for clawing and ECRB to AP transfer for thumb adduction.

- The recommended nerve transfer in ulnar nerve palsy is the distal AIN to ulnar nerve deep motor branch transfer.

DISCLOSURE

The authors have nothing to disclose.

REFERENCES

1. Noble J, Munro CA, Prasad VS, et al. Analysis of upper and lower extremity peripheral nerve injuries in a

population of patients with multiple injuries. J Trauma 1998;45(1):116–22.

2. Lin JS, Jain SA. Challenges in nerve repair and reconstruction. Hand Clin 2023;39(3):403–15.

3. Karsy M, Watkins R, Jensen MR, et al. Trends and cost analysis of upper extremity nerve injury using the National (Nationwide) inpatient sample. World Neurosurg 2019;123:e488–500.

4. Gardenier J, Garg R, Mudgal C. Upper extremity tendon transfers: a brief review of history, common applications, and technical tips. Indian J Plast Surg 2020;53(2):177–90.

5. Gurunluoglu R, Shafighi M, Huemer GM, et al. Carl Nicoladoni (1847-1902): professor of surgery. Ann Surg 2004;239(2):281–92.

6. Seiler JG 3rd, Desai MJ, Payne SH. Tendon transfers for radial, median, and ulnar nerve palsy. J Am Acad Orthop Surg 2013;21(11):675–84.

7. Grzybowski A, Pietrzak K. Tomasz Drobnik (1858-1901). J Neurol 2016;263(3):624–5.

8. Bunnell J, Boyes J. Tendon transfer surgery. Orthop Clin North Am 1970;1(447):e54.

9. Steindler A. Orthopaedic reconstruction work on hand and forearm. New York Med J 1918;108:1117–9.

10. Brand PW, Beach RB, Thompson DE. Relative tension and potential excursion of muscles in the forearm and hand. J Hand Surg Am 1981;6(3):209–19.

11. Rinker B. Nerve transfers in the upper extremity: a practical user's guide. Ann Plast Surg 2015; 74(Suppl 4):S222–8.

12. Harris RI. The treatment of irreparable nerve injuries. Can Med Assoc J 1921;11(11):833–41.

13. Domeshek LF, Novak CB, Patterson JMM, et al. Nerve transfers-A paradigm shift in the reconstructive ladder. Plast Reconstr Surg Glob Open 2019; 7(6):e2290.

14. Nath RK, Mackinnon SE. Nerve transfers in the upper extremity. Hand Clin 2000;16(1):131–9, ix.

15. Tung TH, Mackinnon SE. Nerve transfers: indications, techniques, and outcomes. J Hand Surg Am 2010;35(2):332–41.

16. Sunderland S. A classification of peripheral nerve injuries producing loss of function. Brain 1951;74(4):491–516.

17. Seddon HJ. A classification of nerve injuries. Br Med J 1942;2(4260):237–9.

18. Compton J, Owens J, Day M, et al. Systematic review of tendon transfer versus nerve transfer for the restoration of wrist extension in isolated traumatic radial nerve palsy. J Am Acad Orthop Surg Glob Res Rev 2018;2(4):e001.

19. Patterson JMM, Russo SA, El-Haj M, et al. Radial nerve palsy: nerve transfer versus tendon transfer to restore function. Hand (N Y) 2022;17(6):1082–9.

20. Giuffre JL, Bishop AT, Spinner RJ, et al. The best of tendon and nerve transfers in the upper extremity. Plast Reconstr Surg 2015;135(3):617e–30e.

21. Goyal K, Chepla KJ. Tendon transfers: techniques to minimize complications. Hand Clin 2023;39(3):447–53.

22. Power DM, Mikalef P, Cavallaro DC. A comparison of tendon and nerve transfer surgery for reconstruction of upper limb paralysis. Journal of Musculoskeletal Surgery and Research 2019;3:69–74.

23. Loewenstein SN, Adkinson JM. Tendon transfers for peripheral nerve palsies. Clin Plast Surg 2019;46(3):307–15.

24. Curtis RM. Fundamental principles of tendon transfer. Orthop Clin North Am 1974;5(2):231–42.

25. Sammer DM, Chung KC. Tendon transfers: part I. Principles of transfer and transfers for radial nerve palsy. Plast Reconstr Surg 2009;123(5):169e–77e.

26. Cheah AE, Etcheson J, Yao J. Radial nerve tendon transfers. Hand Clin 2016;32(3):323–38.

27. Horii E, An KN, Linscheid RL. Excursion of prime wrist tendons. J Hand Surg Am 1993;18(1):83–90.

28. Ray WZ, Mackinnon SE. Management of nerve gaps: autografts, allografts, nerve transfers, and end-to-side neurorrhaphy. Exp Neurol 2010;223(1):77–85.

29. Brown JM, Mackinnon SE. Nerve transfers in the forearm and hand. Hand Clin 2008;24(4):319–40.

30. Fox IK, Mackinnon SE. Adult peripheral nerve disorders: nerve entrapment, repair, transfer, and brachial plexus disorders. Plast Reconstr Surg 2011;127(5):105e–18e.

31. Bertelli JA. Nerve versus tendon transfer for radial nerve paralysis reconstruction. J Hand Surg Am 2020;45(5):418–26.

32. Peters BR, Van Handel AC, Russo SA, et al. Five reliable nerve transfers for the treatment of isolated upper extremity nerve injuries. Plast Reconstr Surg 2021;147(5):830e–45e.

33. Davidge KM, Yee A, Kahn LC, et al. Median to radial nerve transfers for restoration of wrist, finger, and thumb extension. J Hand Surg Am 2013;38(9):1812–27.

34. Ray WZ, Mackinnon SE. Clinical outcomes following median to radial nerve transfers. J Hand Surg Am 2011;36(2):201–8.

35. Chuinard RG, Boyes JH, Stark HH, et al. Tendon transfers for radial nerve palsy: use of superficialis tendons for digital extension. J Hand Surg Am 1978;3(6):560–70.

36. Pet MA, Lipira AB, Ko JH. Nerve transfers for the restoration of wrist, finger, and thumb extension after high radial nerve injury. Hand Clin 2016;32(2):191–207.

37. Mackinnon SE, Roque B, Tung TH. Median to radial nerve transfer for treatment of radial nerve palsy. Case report. J Neurosurg 2007;107(3):666–71.

38. Camitz H. Uber die Behandlung der Oppositionslahmung. Acta Chir Scand 1929;65:77–81.

39. Huber E. Hilfsoperation bei median Uhlahmung. Dtsch Arch Klin Med 1921;136:271.

40. Bunnell S. Opposition of the thumb. J Bone Joint Surg 1938;20:269–84.

41. Littler JW, Cooley SG. Opposition of the thumb and its restoration by abductor digiti Quinti transfer. J Bone Joint Surg Am 1963;45:1389–96.

42. Burkhalter W, Christensen RC, Brown P. Extensor indicis proprius opponensplasty. J Bone Joint Surg Am 1973;55(4):725–32.

43. Rymer B, Thomas PB. The Camitz transfer and its modifications: a review. J Hand Surg Eur Vol 2016; 41(6):632–7.

44. Coulshed N, Xu J, Graham D, et al. Opponensplasty for nerve palsy: a systematic review. Hand (N Y) 2023. 15589447231174481.

45. Yavari P, Fadaei B, Ghasemi Darestani N, et al. Comparison of opponensplasty techniques in isolated low median nerve palsy. Int J Burns Trauma 2020; 10(5):263–8.

46. Gottschalk HP, Bindra RR. Late reconstruction of ulnar nerve palsy. Orthop Clin North Am 2012;43(4): 495–507.

47. Tse R, Hentz VR, Yao J. Late reconstruction for ulnar nerve palsy. Hand Clin 2007;23(3):373–92, vii.

48. Sammer DM, Chung KC. Tendon transfers: Part II. Transfers for ulnar nerve palsy and median nerve palsy. Plast Reconstr Surg 2009;124(3):212e–21e.

49. Brand PW. Tendon grafting illustrated by a new operation for intrinsic paralysis of the fingers. J Bone Joint Surg 1961;43B:444–53.

50. Mackinnon SE, Colbert SH. Nerve transfers in the hand and upper extremity surgery. Tech Hand Up Extrem Surg 2008;12(1):20–33.

51. Zancolli EA. Claw-hand caused by paralysis of the intrinsic muscles: a simple surgical procedure for its correction. J Bone Joint Surg Am 1957;39-A(5): 1076–80.

52. Bunnell S. Surgery of the intrinsic muscles of the hand other than those producing opposition of the thumb. J Bone Joint Surg 1942;24:1–3.

53. Davis T. Tendon transfers for median, radial, and ulnar nerve palsy, . Green's operative hand surgery. 8 edition. Elsevier; 2022. p. 1189–242. chap 31.

Proximal and Distal Nerve Transfers in the Management of Brachial Plexus Injuries

Soo Jin Woo, MD[a,b], Johnny Chuieng-Yi Lu, MD, MSCI[b,*]

KEYWORDS

- Brachial plexus injury - Nerve transfer - Nerve graft - FFMT

KEY POINTS

- Brachial plexus injuries pose significant challenges due to their complexity, requiring detailed preoperative evaluation and a multifaceted surgical approach for effective management.
- Preoperative diagnostics, including physical examinations and electrodiagnostic tests, play a pivotal role in determining the injury site and guiding treatment decisions. Accurate classification of injury levels and comprehensive surgical planning, involving both proximal and distal nerve transfers, are crucial for the optimal restoration of function.
- Nerve transfer, a key surgical strategy, utilizes both intraplexus and extraplexus donors, with the choice influenced by the pattern and extent of injury.
- The Chang Gung approach emphasizes the importance of exploration-driven diagnosis, integrating the strengths of both proximal and distal nerve transfers, and preparing for potential failures with backup plans.

PERSPECTIVES ON BRACHIAL PLEXUS RECONSTRUCTION

Challenges in Brachial Plexus Injuries

Adult brachial plexus injuries (BPIs) significantly impair function and quality of life, leading to lifelong disabilities. The complexity of BPIs, involving a network of essential nerves for upper extremity innervation, presents multifaceted challenges, including complex preoperative planning, unpredictable outcomes after surgery, and the need for intensive rehabilitative interventions. In BPIs, the distance from the nerve repair site to the target muscle is longer than in isolated nerve injuries, delaying muscle reinnervation. Additionally, patients often have concurrent injuries such as head trauma, spinal fractures, and thoracic injuries that further delay the timing of nerve reconstruction.[1,2] The delayed regeneration time, exacerbated by the distance needed for reinnervation, leads to inconsistent outcomes that preclude the patient from regaining a functional limb.

The management of BPIs focuses on the pattern and extent of injury to the nerve roots from C5 to T1. In root avulsion injuries, nerves are torn from their intraspinal attachments, resulting in only one disrupted end (distal) with a coiled spring-like appearance in the acute stage or a fusiform pattern in the chronic stage. The proximal nerve end is notably absent, making nerve repair or grafting impossible (**Fig. 1**). Root rupture injuries, on the other hand, result in a complete division

[a] W Institute for Hand and Reconstructive Microsurgery, W General Hospital, 1632 Dalgubeol-daero, Dalseo-gu, Daegu, South Korea; [b] Division of Reconstructive Microsurgery, Department of Plastic Surgery, Chang Gung University, Chang Gung Memorial Hospital, 5 Fu-Hsing Street, Kuei-Shan, Taoyuan 333, Taiwan
* Corresponding author. Division of Reconstructive Microsurgery, Department of Plastic Surgery, Chang Gung University, Chang Gung Memorial Hospital, 5 Fu-Hsing Street, Kuei-Shan, Taoyuan 333, Taiwan.
E-mail address: cylu122@gmail.com

Clin Plastic Surg 51 (2024) 485–494
https://doi.org/10.1016/j.cps.2024.02.014
0094-1298/24/© 2024 Elsevier Inc. All rights reserved.

Avulsion injury

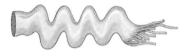

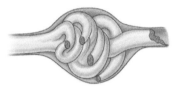

A. Coiled spring-like structure (acute stage)

B. Fusiform pattern neuroma (chronic stage)

Rupture injury

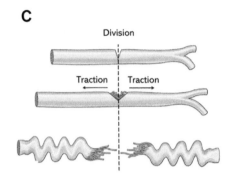

Fig. 1. The underlying mechanisms of avulsion injuries (*A, B*) in contrast to rupture injuries (*C*). (*From*: Chuang DC-C. Brachial plexus injuries: Adult and pediatric. In: Chang J, Neligan PC. Plastic surgery. Volume 6: Hand and Upper Limb. Elsevier Health Sciences. 2017. p. 812–844.)

of the nerve with distinct proximal and distal stumps. These injures are amenable to nerve grafting due to the visibility of nerve ends within the operative field. Unfortunately, avulsions occur in up to 89% of cases,[1,3] with a significant 26% involving all 5 roots,[4] necessitating nerve transfers to restore distal nerve function.

Understanding another critical component of BPIs involves classifying the level of injury. Traditional perspectives categorize injury levels into 2 groups: (1) preganglionic versus postganglionic root injuries and (2) supraclavicular versus infraclavicular injuries. Injuries to the root may be unpredictable, potentially affecting parts or the entirety of the dorsal and ventral rootlets; extensive injuries may involve both the intraspinal and extraspinal levels simultaneously. These perspectives render the division of injury level into preganglionic and postganglionic categories impractical, necessitating a more functional classification. An example of this is Chuang's classification,[5] which categorizes injury levels as I (inside the vertebral bone: avulsed and ungraftable), II (inside the scalene muscle: ruptured and graftable), III (preclavicular and retroclavicular), and IV (infraclavicular). Classifying the level of injury in this manner aids in deciding the type of nerve reconstruction and provides a uniform platform for all team members to communicate using a common language.

NERVE TRANSFER FOR BRACHIAL PLEXUS INJURIES

Nerve transfer is a surgical strategy that uses an available and expendable donor nerve and transferring it to a recipient nerve. It has emerged as a

pivotal technique in managing BPIs, underpinned by historical contributions such as those by Harris and Low in 1903, who pioneered the idea of suturing the distal stump of a damaged spinal nerve to a neighboring healthy nerve.[6] The routine use of various nerve transfers has transformed the landscape of BPI management and recovery. It is recognized that the procedure performs optimally within a definitive timeframe, preferably within 6 months after the injury, to effectively reactivate the paralyzed muscles. While nomenclature may vary, nerve transfers can be broadly classified into proximal and distal nerve transfers[7] based on the distance from the nerve coaptation site to the neuromuscular junction, the scar encountered during dissection, and whether the recipient nerve branches out distally.[8] In the following sections, we will detail the specific types of nerve transfers, with focus on reinnervation of shoulder reinnervation and elbow flexion (**Table 1**).

Proximal Nerve Transfers

Proximal nerve transfers include intraplexus and extraplexus nerve transfers. Intraplexus nerve transfer is applicable in cases of incomplete BPIs, where at least one of the spinal nerves remains intact. However, in situations of complete root avulsions, the use of intraplexus donor nerves becomes unfeasible, necessitating reliance on extraplexus donors from the ipsilateral or contralateral neck. Notable extraplexus donor nerve options include the phrenic nerve, deep cervical motor branches, hypoglossal nerve, spinal accessory nerve (XI), intercostal nerve (ICN), and the contralateral C7 (CC7) spinal nerve.[5] Esteemed experts like Narakas, Millesi, Gilbert, Terzis, and

Table 1
Nerve transfer approaches in cases of brachial plexus injury with increased arsenal of donor nerves after neck exploration

	Shoulder	Elbow	Wrist Extension	Fingers
C5-C6, C5-C7 injury with intact triceps	• Ph/XI to SS • Triceps to Ax • C5 to PD of UT	• <u>C7 PD to AD of UT</u>	—	—
C5-C7 injury without triceps	• Ph/XI to SS • ICN to Ax • C5/XI to PD of UT	• <u>Branch of UN/MN to MCN</u> • ICN to triceps	—	—
C5-C8 injury with intact wrist extension	• Ph/XI to SS • ICN to Ax • M. Pec to Ax • C5/XI to PD of UT	• <u>Branch of UN/MN to MCN</u> • ICN to triceps	—	—
C5-C8 injury without wrist extension	• Ph/XI to SS • ICN to Ax • C5/XI to PD of UT	• <u>Branch of UN/MN to MCN</u> • ICN to triceps	• AION PQ to ECRB • Wrist arthrodesis	—
C5-T1 injury with C5 rupture	• Ph to SS • ICN to Ax	• <u>C5 to MCN and MN by VUNG</u> • ICN to triceps	• Wrist arthrodesis	• C5 to MCN and MN by VUNG
C5-T1 injury with total root avulsion	• <u>Ph to SS</u>	• <u>ICN to MCN</u>	• Wrist arthrodesis	• CC7 to MN by VUNG

Underlined text indicates the primary preferred nerve transfer strategy.

Abbreviations: Ph, phrenic nerve; XI, spinal accessory nerve; SS, suprascapular nerve; Ax, axillary nerve; PD, posterior division; UT, upper trunk; AD, anterior division; ICN, intercostal nerve; UN, ulnar nerve; MN, median nerve; MCN, musculocutaneous nerve; M.Pec, medial pectoral nerve; AION PQ, anterior interosseous nerve to pronator quadratus; ECRB, extensor carpi radialis brevis; VUNG, vascularized ulnar nerve graft; CC7, contralateral C7.

Chuang have traditionally endorsed this approach, with an emphasis on exploring the injured plexus to (1) diagnose and (2) explore for viable donor nerves. If preoperative examination shows evidence that a ruptured spinal nerve is highly likely, it is imperative to not waste this source of viable axons. In adult BPIs, upper roots are more prone to rupture, underscoring the need for proximal exploration. The lower roots, in contrast, are more likely to be avulsed.[9] For proximal nerve transfers, nerve grafts are frequently required to connect healthy proximal and distal stumps to facilitate reinnervation. Commonly used autografts include sural nerves, sensory nerves from the paralyzed arm such as the radial sensory nerve and medial antebrachial cutaneous nerves, and vascularized ulnar nerve grafts (VUNGs) when both C8 and T1 roots are avulsed.[10]

C5 (or other viable roots) nerve grafting to divisions of the upper trunk for the elbow and/or shoulder

The benefits of grafting the ruptured spinal nerves to the division or trunk level for elbow or shoulder are as follows: (1) restoring the natural pathway, (2) lack of donor nerve morbidities involving the median or ulnar nerve, (3) ease of rehabilitation for patients that lack understanding of induction exercise,[11] and (4) potential for ongoing functional improvement after initial years of surgery, which is less common with distal nerve transfer. The disadvantages include longer rehabilitation time and the unpredictability of regeneration across nerve grafts. Nerve grafting is not ideal in patients who present more than 6 months from injury, have gaps more than 6 cm, are aged older than 50 years. Additionally, nerve grafting is particularly suboptimal in the restoration of elbow flexion.[12]

C5 or contralateral C7 to musculocutaneous and median nerve via free vascularized ulnar nerve graft for the elbow and hand

VUNG is indicated to bridge long nerve gaps (>10 cm) with an underlying scarred wound bed (**Fig. 2**). While prior studies have cited inconsistent outcomes with the use of pedicled VUNG in total root avulsion,[13,14] our institute has modified this method by using free VUNG.[10] In pan-plexus

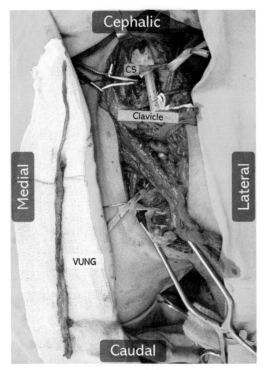

Fig. 2. Intraoperative view demonstrating the use of a VUNG to span a nerve defect over 10 cm, linking the C5 nerve to the musculocutaneous nerve.

palsy, the goal is to connect a healthy donor stump at the root level to important target nerves close to the target muscles, such as the musculocutaneous nerve (MCN) or median nerve. C5 is an ideal donor option when found ruptured, while the CC7 is indicated in cases of total root avulsion. The CC7 is a robust donor owing to its rich composition of healthy myelinated nerve fibers with abundance of axons and acceptable donor nerve morbidity.[15] Our recent study suggests that VUNG from the ipsilateral C5 can provide sufficient elbow flexion and finger flexion even when VUNG is connected to 2 targets; in contrast, CC7 is more suitable for a single target.[16]

C7 posterior division to anterior division of upper trunk transfer for the elbow

After introducing the CC7 nerve root transfer in 1991,[13] Gu proposed the use of the ipsilateral C7 to address C5 ruptures in 2003.[15] When C5, C6 roots are avulsed, the posterior division (PD) of the ipsilateral C7 is a powerful donor nerve that can be coapted primarily to anterior division (AD) of upper trunk (UT) to restore elbow flexion. The PD of C7 encompasses 66.2% of all the motor fibers originating from C7, ensuring adequate motive power for functional improvement.[17] A significant benefit of this procedure is that it can be

conducted through a single supraclavicular incision, facilitating both exploration and repair. This transfer restores anterior shoulder flexion through the reinnervation of the clavicular head of the pectoralis major, though this may also inadvertently counter shoulder abduction.

Spinal accessory or phrenic nerve grafting to musculocutaneous nerve for the elbow

In root avulsion injuries when intraplexus donors are not available, extraplexus donors such as XI or phrenic nerve are alternative options. Both can be reliably coapted to the AD of UT primarily. Size mismatch and potential for misrouting axons to unwanted targets warrants selection of a more distal target. Socolovsky and colleagues compared coapting to (1) AD of UT with a shorter graft or (2) MCN with longer nerve grafts and found that coapting to AD lead to axonal misrouting in 25% of cases, while length of graft did not affect the final outcome.[18]

Distal Nerve Transfers

Distal nerve transfers provide an appealing alternative to proximal nerve transfers by employing both expendable extraplexal and intraplexal sources in incomplete injuries, thereby expanding the available options. Distal transfers involve coaptation sites located closer to the target organ, which can be muscle or skin, and are thus referred to as close-target nerve transfers. These techniques are usually performed in nonscarred areas and typically utilize a branch or fascicle of a healthy nerve (eg, the pronator quadratus branch of the anterior interosseous nerve) to innervate the major terminal branch of a critically injured nerve (eg, the deep motor branch of the ulnar nerve). Advantages include quicker reinnervation, less misrouting of donor axons, and direct nerve coaptation without the need for nerve grafts.[9] Exploration at the site of injury is not a prerequisite for distal nerve transfers, but it is still warranted to confirm the diagnosis prior to reconstruction. Incorrect diagnosis without dissection could exacerbate situations such as incomplete injuries or compression neuropathies and lead to unnecessary nerve transfers.

Oberlin-I and Mackinnon nerve transfer for the elbow

The focus of these transfers is to directly reinnervate the biceps and/or brachialis branch of the MCN, thereby bypassing the scarred region in the proximal plexus, and avoiding misrouting. Indications include C5-6, C5-7, and/or C5-8 injury when patients still demonstrate acceptable wrist and finger flexion. A variety of donor nerves including the nerve fascicle to flexor carpi ulnaris

(FCU; Oberlin-I),[19] FCU and flexor digitorum superficialis (FDS; double fascicular transfer),[20] median pectoral, thoracodorsal, spinal accessory, and ICNs, have been reported for this purpose.

The Oberlin-I transfer method entails the reallocation of fascicles from the ulnar nerve to the bicep's motor nerve.[19] The Mackinnon transfer is a double fascicular transfer involving expendable fascicles from the median and ulnar nerves.[20] Both transfers are primarily indicated when there is a lack of elbow flexion but preserved hand and wrist function. Contraindications include weakness or absence of wrist flexion or FDS, indicating inadequate donor nerve availability. Numerous studies have engaged in comparative analyses of the Oberlin and Mackinnon transfers, sparking a debate over their relative efficacy. Some reports found no significant difference in outcomes between the 2 methods,[21] while certain meta-analyses suggest a subtle superiority of Mackinnon transfers when performed within 6 months postinjury.[22] Our center's results show a definitive superiority of the Mackinnon transfer over Oberlin-I in C5-6 patients and in patients who underwent delayed surgical intervention.[23]

Intercostal to musculocutaneous nerve transfer for the elbow

Intercostal to MCN transfer was initially introduced by Chiasserini in 1934 for paraplegics.[24] It has since become instrumental in restoring elbow flexion following total nerve root avulsions in BPIs. ICN transfers have effectively restored elbow flexion, with 87% of patients achieving an Medical Research Council (MRC) grade 3 or above.[25] The ideal number of donor ICNs to use is still under debate. Our previous study showed evidence that using 3 ICNs is optimal due to the increased axon count and better diameter matching with the musculocutaneous.[26] After ICN transfer procedures, patients are advised to restrict passive shoulder elevation to less than 90° for 6 months and ensure regular follow-ups at the rehabilitation center. Respiratory exercises such as climbing stairs are important to stimulate the donor nerve. This can be combined with deep breathing and deliberate full exhalation. Poor outcomes are more often seen in elderly patients, heavy smokers, or severely obese patients. Concerns may arise regarding the availability of ICN transfer, especially given that thoracic cavity injuries like pneumothorax or rib fractures are present in 25% to 52% of patients with BPIs.[1,2] Yet, a 92% success rate was achieved even in those with concurrent chest trauma. Rib fractures were not a significant complication factor, although rib fractures were noted to affect nerve viability.[27]

Spinal accessory or phrenic nerve to suprascapular nerve transfer for the shoulder

Regaining shoulder function is a central objective in managing upper BPIs, second only to the restoration of elbow flexion. Functional shoulder abduction, essential for reaching objects, is initiated by the supraspinatus muscle (0°–60°) and augmented by the deltoid muscle (60°–180°), with the suprascapular and axillary nerves providing innervation, respectively. Additionally, the stability of the shoulder girdle, which is crucial for functional shoulder movement, depends on the serratus anterior, trapezius, levator scapulae, and rhomboid muscles. To restore shoulder stability, external rotation, and abduction, recovery efforts focus on reinnervating the distal C5, suprascapular nerve, PD of the UT, and then the axillary nerve, in that order of priority.

In our treatment of multiple root BPIs, the transfer from either the spinal accessory nerve or the phrenic nerve to the suprascapular nerve is commonly used to restore shoulder abduction. Both can be accessed during the supraclavicular dissection, with the spinal accessory nerve identified on the anterior surface of the trapezius muscle. The phrenic nerve has emerged as an alternative (**Fig. 3**). Its continuous activation

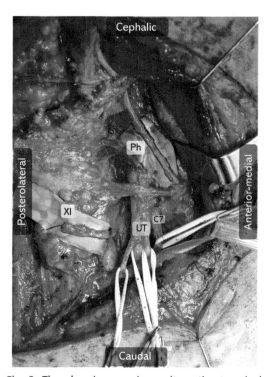

Fig. 3. The phrenic nerve is an alternative to spinal accessory nerve for neurotization of distal targets such as suprascapular nerve. Ph, phrenic nerve; UT, upper trunk; XI, spinal accessory nerve.

through breathing offers consistent induction, even during sleep and regular activities.[28] Additionally, the phrenic nerve has sufficient axon count to restore elbow flexion and shoulder abduction.[29] However, phrenic nerve is controversial due to the potential for permanent ipsilateral diaphragm paralysis, affecting pulmonary function. Various studies indicate that patients generally tolerate postoperative symptoms, and most patients see improvements in respiratory distress within a period ranging from 6 months to 2 years after surgery.[28] In practice, its application must consider patient-specific factors such as age, pre-existing respiratory pathologies, and high body mass index.

Our recent study demonstrated that patients who underwent phrenic nerve transfer achieved outcomes in maximum shoulder abduction comparable to those with the XI transfer.[29] Given its easier accessibility during routine supraclavicular plexus exploration, our preference is to use the phrenic nerve for shoulder, while preserving the XI for secondary reconstruction such as functioning free muscle transplantation (FFMT).

Triceps or medial pectoral branch to axillary nerve transfer for the shoulder

The triceps branch of radial nerve and the medial pectoral nerve transfer to axillary nerve transfer are 2 donor options to reinnervate the deltoid muscle.[30] For the triceps branch to axillary nerve transfer, it is essential to have intact triceps function, which can be found in isolated axillary nerve or C5-6 BPIs. Both the branch to the long head of triceps[31] and medial head of triceps[32] are reliable donors. Targeting the anterior branch of the axillary nerve is sufficient to achieve full range of motion in shoulder abduction.[31]

On the other hand, the medial pectoral nerve from the lower trunk (C8-T1) is used for cases with weak or absent triceps function stemming from C5-7 injury. This is not advisable when the sternal head of the pectoralis major muscle is denervated, such as C5-8 injury or pan-plexus BPI. Of note, the medial pectoral nerve has limitations due to its length, diameter mismatch, and antagonistic function of the shoulder adduction.[33]

Intercostal nerve to axillary nerve transfer for the shoulder and/or triceps branch of radial nerve for elbow extension

Due to the availability of multiple ICNs that can be harvested for transfer to the axillary region, it is possible to harvest third and fourth ICNs for axillary nerve (anterior branch) and then fifth and sixth ICNs for triceps branch of radial nerve. Using the ICN in the context of limb extension is compatible

and easier for the patient to train. Indications include pan-plexus or C5-8 injury where the proximal roots are avulsed. ICNs to MCN should not be performed simultaneously, as these can be antagonistic to elbow movement. Phrenic to suprascapular nerve transfer combined with ICNs to axillary nerve transfer is a feasible combination in young, eager patients without previously mentioned contraindications.

Long thoracic nerve reinnervation for shoulder

The long thoracic nerve adds to shoulder stability through its innervation of the serratus anterior muscle. The XI, ICNs, and medial branch of the thoracodorsal nerve are potential donors. The selection of a nerve for transfer is strategically made based on the specific roots injured and the requirement for improved scapular stabilization and protraction.

The Chang Gung Approach in Brachial Plexus Injuries

The Chang Gung philosophy toward managing BPIs emphasizes the importance of exploration, subsequently incorporating both proximal and distal nerve transfers, while always maintaining a backup strategy. Exploration of the neck is an indispensable step: "no exploration, no diagnosis, no surgery." This becomes particularly critical when a C5 rupture might be mistakenly interpreted as a root avulsion.[34] A healthy C5 stump can serve as a robust mother nerve with an abundance of axons and power and eliminates the need for unnecessary distal nerve transfers. While distal nerve transfer surgeries have become standard for BPIs and other high-level peripheral nerve injuries, the Chang Gung approach continues to prioritize proximal transfers as the main reconstructive method, based on the principle of exploration-driven diagnosis. Distal nerve transfers offer only surgical intervention and should not replace proximal nerve transfers when the latter is indicated. The authors wish to emphasize that proximal nerve transfers not only provide a more accurate diagnosis but also facilitate proper treatment, restoring both shoulder and elbow functions concurrently. On the other hand, distal nerve transfers have the potential to yield more efficient elbow flexion. Therefore, when faced with scenarios where there is either an absence of a healthy donor nerve or an insufficient one, the authors advocate for the combination of both strategies as the preferred method of primary nerve reconstruction.

Recent literature has compared distal and proximal nerve transfers. In our study involving a cohort of 147 patients undergoing various MCN techniques, the elbow flexion recovery rate showed no significant difference between proximal and distal nerve transfers.[35] The distal group recovered slightly faster at 19 months compared to 23.9 months for the proximal group, though this was not statistically significant.[35] Since both techniques have their unique advantages and limitations, the decision on which would be more beneficial should be based on the patient's specific condition and the surgeon's expertise. It is imperative that surgeons master the skill of exploration to ensure that the option of proximal nerve transfer is always available. By integrating the strengths of both proximal and distal nerve transfers, patients benefit from correct diagnosis, availability of multiple donors, and faster target reinnervation.

ADDRESSING FAILURES AND ESTABLISHING BACKUPS
Decision-making Process

Recognizing potential failures and planning backups in nerve transfer procedures is paramount. A proactive and systematic approach can significantly improve outcomes and minimize the

adverse effects of unsuccessful surgeries. A failed nerve transfer becomes evident when deformities persist after an extended period of recovery. Given this delayed manifestation of potential failures, the initial surgical intervention must be executed with the foresight of potential setbacks, ensuring avenues remain open for subsequent treatments. This necessitates the meticulous preservation of available donor nerves and vessels during primary surgeries. For example, if a pan-plexus patient presents more than 6 months after injury and is at high risk for failure, the surgeon should be mindful to preserve at least one donor nerve such as the ICNs for backup FFMT reinnervation.[23]

For effective decision-making, comprehensive documentation is mandatory (**Fig. 4**). The BPI presents in intricate and diverse ways. While it is a given that preoperative histories and findings from clinical examinations must be accurately recorded, it is equally critical to maintain detailed and individualized intraoperative records for the formulation of a robust backup plan. Doing so captures the nature of injuries, procedures conducted, and the status of structures whether retained or

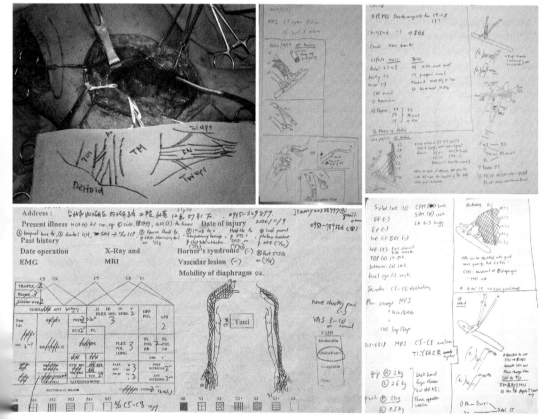

Fig. 4. A collection of documents illustrating comprehensive patient history taking, neurologic examination, preoperative planning, surgical details and postoperative follow-up, emphasizing the importance of thorough documentation for patients with BPI.

sacrificed. This documentation not only facilitates the refinement of future interventions but also ensures that care remains adaptive and tailored to each patient.

Palliative Procedures

FFMT has emerged as a popular option for late-presenting BPI cases, especially when conventional nerve surgeries have either failed or been delayed. Primarily, it is indicated to restore elbow function, particularly when the time from injury to surgery exceeds 9 to 12 months.[36] In cases of total root avulsion, the debate over prioritizing multiple nerve transfers versus FFMT reconstruction is ongoing.[9] However, our approach is inclined toward using FFMT as a secondary adjuvant reconstruction to enhance outcomes at a later stage.

Other backup plans encompass palliative reconstruction procedures such as tendon transfers, arthrodesis, the alternative use of orthotics, or in some cases, amputation combined with prosthetics. Tendon transfers can augment a range of upper limb functions for patients with passively supple and mobile joints. The efficacy of these transfers largely depends on the presence of muscles unaffected by injury, which can act as donor muscles. For instance, the trapezius muscle, being innervated by the spinal accessory nerve, is a favorable choice for muscle transfer to improve external rotation.[37] Shoulder fusion is considered, to enhance limb stability, when addressing a subluxated shoulder with poor shoulder reinnervation.[38] Meanwhile, wrist fusion can enhance the efficacy of free-functioning muscle transfers for grasp.[39]

SUMMARY

In managing BPIs, nerve transfer techniques encompass various methods, including both proximal and distal approaches, selected based on injury patterns and nerve availability. The Chang Gung approach recommends a strategy that combines proximal and distal nerve transfers, guided by exploration-driven diagnosis, to achieve optimal functional recovery, while also emphasizing the importance of having contingency plans for potential surgical failures.

CLINICS CARE POINTS

- Exploration-driven diagnosis: Emphasize the importance of detailed exploration of the brachial plexus to accurately diagnose the extent of injury, crucial for guiding subsequent surgical decisions.

- Prioritization of proximal transfers: While integrating both proximal and distal nerve transfers, prioritize proximal transfers based on their potential for restoring shoulder and elbow functions concurrently.

- Backup strategies: Always maintain a backup plan, including alternative nerve transfer options, to address potential failures of the initial surgical intervention.

- Integration of techniques: Combine the strengths of both proximal and distal nerve transfers to benefit from accurate diagnosis, multiple donor options, and faster target reinnervation.

- Tailored surgical intervention: Customize nerve transfer strategies based on the patient's specific condition, ensuring that surgical choices are guided by both exploratory findings and the surgeon's expertise.

DISCLOSURE

The authors declare that there are no conflicts of interest, financial or otherwise, that could influence or bias the content of this study.

REFERENCES

1. Jain DKA, Bhardwaj P, Venkataramani H, et al. An epidemiological study of traumatic brachial plexus injury patients treated at an Indian centre. Indian J Plast Surg 2012;45(03):498–503.
2. Kaiser R, Mencl L, Haninec P. Injuries associated with serious brachial plexus involvement in poly-trauma among patients requiring surgical repair. Injury 2014;45(1):223–6.
3. Songcharoen P. Brachial plexus injury in Thailand: a report of 520 cases. Microsurgery 1995;16(1):35–9.
4. Kaiser R, Waldauf P, Ullas G, et al. Epidemiology, etiology, and types of severe adult brachial plexus injuries requiring surgical repair: systematic review and meta-analysis. Neurosurg Rev 2020;43:443–52.
5. Chuang DC-C. Brachial plexus injury: nerve reconstruction and functioning muscle transplantation. Semin Plast Surg 2010;057–66.
6. Harris W, Low VW. On the importance of accurate muscular analysis in lesions of the brachial plexus and the treatment of Erb's palsy and infantile paralysis of the upper extremity by cross-union of the nerve roots. Br Med J 1903;1035–8.
7. Chuang DC-C. Brachial plexus injuries: adult and pediatric. In: Chang J, Neligan PC, editors. Plastic surgery. Hand and upper limb, ume 6. Elsevier Health Sciences; 2017. p. 812–44.
8. Chuang DC-C. Distal nerve transfers: a perspective on the future of reconstructive microsurgery. J Reconstr Microsurg 2018;34(09):669–71.

9. Lu JC-Y, Chuang DC-C. Adult brachial plexus injuries: a historical perspective. In: Shin AY, Pulos N, editors. Operative brachial plexus surgery: clinical evaluation and management strategies. Springer; 2021. p. 1–15.

10. Chuang DC-C, Wei F-C, Noordhoff MS. Cross-chest C7 nerve grafting followed by free muscle transplantations for the treatment of total avulsed brachial plexus injuries: a preliminary report. Plast Reconstr Surg 1993;92(4):717–25.

11. Chuang DC-C. Nerve transfers in adult brachial plexus injuries: my methods. Hand Clin 2005;21(1): 71–82.

12. Lin JT-K, Lee Y-H, Lee C-H, et al. What makes nerve grafting work in brachial plexus injuries: a multivariate and survival analysis of commonly affiliated variables. J Plast Reconstr Aesthet Surg 2023;76: 51–3.

13. Gu Y-d, Zhang G-m, Chen D-s, et al. Cervical nerve root transfer from contralateral normal side for treatment of brachial plexus root avulsions. Chin Med J (Engl). 1991;104(03):208–11.

14. Bertelli JA, Ghizoni MF. Nerve root grafting and distal nerve transfers for C5-C6 brachial plexus injuries. J Hand Surg Am 2010;35(5):769–75.

15. Gu YD, Cai PQ, Xu F, et al. Clinical application of ipsilateral C7 nerve root transfer for treatment of C5 and C6 avulsion of brachial plexus. Microsurgery 2003;23(2):105–8.

16. Lin JA-J, Lu JC-Y, Chang TN-J, et al. Long-term outcome of 118 acute total brachial plexus injury patients using free vascularized ulnar nerve graft to innervate the median nerve. J Reconstr Microsurg 2022;39(04):279–87.

17. Huang X, You Z, Xiang Y, et al. Posterior division of ipsilateral C7 transfer to C5 for shoulder abduction limitation. Front Neurol 2023;14:1012977.

18. Socolovsky M, Di Masi G, Battaglia D. Use of long autologous nerve grafts in brachial plexus reconstruction: factors that affect the outcome. Acta Neurochir 2011;153:2231–40.

19. Oberlin C, Beal D, Leechavengvongs S, et al. Nerve transfer to biceps muscle using a part of ulnar nerve for C5–C6 avulsion of the brachial plexus: anatomical study and report of four cases. J Hand Surg Am 1994;19(2):232–7.

20. Mackinnon SE, Novak CB, Myckatyn TM, et al. Results of reinnervation of the biceps and brachialis muscles with a double fascicular transfer for elbow flexion. J Hand Surg Am 2005;30(5):978–85.

21. Martins RS, Siqueira MG, Heise CO, et al. A prospective study comparing single and double fascicular transfer to restore elbow flexion after brachial plexus injury. Neurosurgery 2013;72(5): 709–15.

22. Donnelly MR, Rezzadeh KT, Vieira D, et al. Is one nerve transfer enough? A systematic review and pooled analysis comparing ulnar fascicular nerve transfer and double ulnar and median fascicular nerve transfer for restoration of elbow flexion after traumatic brachial plexus injury. Microsurgery 2020;40(3):361–9.

23. Wong A, Lee Y-H, Chang TN-J, et al. Delayed nerve reconstruction for brachial plexus injuries: is the risk worth the reward? J Neurosurg 2023;1(aop): 1–8.

24. Chiasserini A. Tentativi di cura in casi di paraplegia da lesione de midollo lombare consecutiva a frattura vertebrale (anastomosi radiculo-intercostale). Il Policlinico 1934;12:603–7.

25. Nagano A, Yamamoto S, Mikami Y. Intercostal nerve transfer to restore upper extremity functions after brachial plexus injury. Ann Acad Med Singap 1995;24(4 Suppl):42–5.

26. Chuang DC-C, Yeh M-C, Wei F-C. Intercostal nerve transfer of the musculocutaneous nerve in avulsed brachial plexus injuries: evaluation of 66 patients. J Hand Surg Am 1992;17(5):822–8.

27. Kovachevich R, Kircher MF, Wood CM, et al. Complications of intercostal nerve transfer for brachial plexus reconstruction. J Hand Surg Am 2010; 35(12):1995–2000.

28. Chuang M-L, Chuang DC-C, Lin I-F, et al. Ventilation and exercise performance after phrenic nerve and multiple intercostal nerve transfers for avulsed brachial plexus injury. Chest 2005; 128(5):3434–9.

29. Lu JC-Y, Lin JA-J, Lee C-H, et al. Phrenic nerve as an alternative donor for nerve transfer to restore shoulder abduction in severe multiple root injuries of the adult brachial plexus. J Hand Surg Am 2023;48(9):954. e1–e954. e10.

30. O'Brien AL, Dengler J, Moore AM. Nerve transfers to shoulder and elbow. In: Shin AY, Pulos N, editors. Operative brachial plexus surgery: clinical evaluation and management strategies. Springer; 2021. p. 163–79.

31. Leechavengvongs S, Witoonchart K, Uerpairojkit C, et al. Nerve transfer to deltoid muscle using the nerve to the long head of the triceps, part II: a report of 7 cases. J Hand Surg Am 2003;28(4):633–8.

32. Novak CB, Mackinnon SE. Distal anterior interosseous nerve transfer to the deep motor branch of the ulnar nerve for reconstruction of high ulnar nerve injuries. J Reconstr Microsurg 2002;18(06): 459–64.

33. Bulstra LF, Shin AY. Nerve transfers to restore elbow function. Hand Clin 2016;32(2):165–74.

34. Yeow Y-J, Yeow K-M, Su I-H, et al. Predicting healthy C5 spinal nerve stumps eligible for grafting with MRI, tinel test, and rhomboid electromyography: a retrospective study of 295 consecutive brachial plexus surgeries. Radiology 2021;300(1): 141–51.

35. Hu C-H, Chang TN-J, Lu JC-Y, et al. Comparison of surgical strategies between proximal nerve graft and/or nerve transfer and distal nerve transfer based on functional restoration of elbow flexion: a retrospective review of 147 patients. Plast Reconstr Surg 2018;141(1):68e–79e.

36. Doi K, Kuwata N, Muramatsu K, et al. Double muscle transfer for upper extremity reconstruction following complete avulsion of the brachial plexus. Hand Clin 1999;15(4):757–67.

37. Aziz W, Singer RM, Wolff TW. Transfer of the trapezius for flail shoulder after brachial plexus injury. J Bone Joint Surg Br 1990;72(4):701–4.

38. Rouholamin E, Wootton J, Jamieson A. Arthrodesis of the shoulder following brachial plexus injury. Injury 1991;22(4):271–4.

39. Addosooki A, Doi K, Hattori Y, et al. Role of wrist arthrodesis in patients receiving double free muscle transfers for reconstruction following complete brachial plexus paralysis. J Hand Surg Am 2012;37(2):277–81.

The Mangled Upper Extremity–Algorithm for Salvage: My Workhorse Flaps

Tsz Kit Kevin Chan, MD[a],*, Kevin C. Chung, MD[b]

KEYWORDS

• Flaps • Mangled hand • Microsurgery • Open fracture

KEY POINTS

- Mangling injuries of the upper extremity are devastating, high-energy, complex traumas requiring broad knowledge in orthopedic, vascular, and plastic surgery. .
- Surgeons need to remain vigilant for other injuries that can threaten a patient's life before attending to the upper extremity.
- General principles of management are (1) aggressive initial debridement to convert a contaminated wound into a clean-contaminated, (2) obtain rigid, bony fixation, (3) restoration of good vascularity, and (4) obtain early (<72 hours) soft tissue coverage when possible.

INTRODUCTION

Mangling injuries of the upper extremity are severe traumas that impart significant disability. They are broadly defined as high-energy injuries affecting multiple functional systems in the hand and upper extremity, including skin/soft tissues, vascular, nerve, tendon, and bone.[1] A "preferred treatment" is not possible due to the innumerable combination of injury patterns and severity. The purposes of this article are to reinforce treatment principles and make recommendations on judgment and timing.

A variety of mechanisms can cause mangling upper extremity injuries. They are usually high energy and can include motor vehicle accidents, industrial, farming, firearms, and explosives. They are often visually alarming, but it is critical to remember the mantra, "life before limb." Address any concerns with airway, breathing, and circulation prior to the mangled extremity. Surgeons need to consider other acute injuries that threaten a patient's life. They must also evaluate the overall injury burden and predict future function to formulate a treatment plan with short- and long-term objectives. Mangled upper extremity injuries are multi-system in nature and demand broad knowledge and familiarity with various techniques in orthopedics, vascular, and plastic surgery.[1] The optimal management of mangled upper extremities is therefore one of the most challenging aspects of hand surgery.

Defining Treatment Goals

The function of the hand is summarized as prehension, or the ability to grasp and manipulate objects.[2] When formulating a reconstructive plan for challenging mutilating hand injuries, it is useful to remember the basic hand functions. These include precision pinch, oppositional pinch, key pinch, chuck grip, hook grip, power grasp, and span grasp.[2] However, when assessing the effects of hand trauma on function, it may be helpful to think of 2 major hand motions instead of 7–that is, thumb-finger pinch and digitopalmar grip. Additionally, it may be useful to think of the hand as 4

[a] Department of Orthopedic Surgery, The University of Michigan Health System, 2098 South Main Street, Ann Arbor, MI 48103-5827, USA; [b] Department of Plastic Surgery, The University of Michigan Health System, 1500 E Medical Drive, Ann Arbor, MI 48103, USA
* Corresponding author. Department of Orthopedic Surgery, The University of Michigan Health System, 24 Frank Lloyd Wright Drive, Lobby A, Suite 1200, Ann Arbor, MI 48106.
E-mail address: chantkk@med.umich.edu

Clin Plastic Surg 51 (2024) 495–503
https://doi.org/10.1016/j.cps.2024.02.015

functional units: (1) opposable thumb, (2) index and middle fingers serve as fixed posts for pinch and power, (3) ring and small fingers act as mobile units of the hand, and (4) the wrist.[1]

In its most basic form then, the hand requires a stable wrist and at least 2 opposable digits with some power.[2] One needs to be a stable post, and the other needs to be mobile to pinch and grasp. There also needs to be a cleft between the digits to accommodate objects. The digits need to be sensate and pain-free. The implication of these concepts is that fewer but functional digits may sometimes provide adequate functional restoration.[3] It has been previously recommended that immediate amputation be performed when 4 of the 6 basic digital parts (bone, joint, skin, tendon, nerve, and vessel) are injured.[2] Other relative indications for amputation include a severely mangled single or border digit, segmental injury, severe contamination, significant articular injury, medical instability or comorbidities preventing lengthy surgery, self-inflicted injury, and/or prolonged ischemia time.[4] While it can be agonizing for the hand surgeon to consider the functional loss caused by amputations, it is worth remembering the incredible plasticity of the hand and its core functions. Heroic attempts to salvage severely injured fingers may lead to painful, stiff, and/or insensate digits, ultimately prolonging patient's functional recovery.

The reconstruction of mangling upper extremity injuries inevitably leads to scar formation. The "one wound–one scar" concept[5] combined with the multi-system nature of these injuries mean that scar will form from the skin down through bone. It is for these reasons that function is so at risk.[1] Minimizing the deleterious effects of scar formation mandates the following general principles: (1) aggressive, complete debridement of devitalized tissue, (2) rigid bony fixation, (3) restoration of good vascularity, and (4) early (<72 hours) soft tissue coverage.

Initial Evaluation

Follow advanced trauma life support protocol and look beyond obvious extremity injuries to address airway, breathing, and circulation issues before the hand and upper extremity. Once stabilized, arguably the most emergent initial management is controlling hemorrhage. We agree with other authors[6] that a tourniquet should be avoided unless direct pressure for 10 minutes does not provide hemostasis. On arrival at the hospital, the wounds may be hemostatic due to thrombus formation. A pressure bandage can be an additional maneuver to control hemorrhage.

Due to the distracting nature of mangled upper extremity injuries (**Fig. 1**), the initial evaluation of these patients needs to be focused and efficient. Pertinent history information include the "when," "where," and "how" of the injury.[1] The time of injury is important in determining ischemia time in dysvascular limbs. Generally accepted warm ischemia times are 12 hours for digits and 6 hours for more proximal injuries due to the higher metabolic demands of muscle.[7] Cold ischemia times can be doubled. However, these are not absolute as replantation has been successfully reported in the digit up to 94 hours and up to 54 hours in the hand[8,9]. The location of injury may impact treatment decisions based on type and severity of contamination. For example, a farming injury is concerning for high levels of contamination and could dictate both the timing of surgical intervention and an aggressive surgical debridement.[1] Finally, the mechanism of injury can help determine the amount of energy imparted on the limb by the injury, and subsequently the "zone of injury" to anticipate and treat.[1] Additional information that may impact surgical decision-making are age, hand dominance, occupation, medical comorbidities, and patient preferences.

The physical examination of patients with severe upper extremity injuries is often difficult because of multiple factors including pain, resuscitation efforts, and other concurrent injuries. However, assessing the limb's vascular status is critical in deciding on the urgency of surgical intervention. The surgeon should inspect the limb for color and skin turgor. The surgeon should palpate for temperature of the limb, and the brachial, radial and ulnar pulses. The capillary refill should be 1 to 2 seconds. The dorsal paronychial skin may be more reliable for capillary refill than the nail bed.[1] A handheld Doppler can also be used when the palpation of distal pulses is equivocal. We also recommend the routine use of pulse oximetry to objectively quantify the amount of distal tissue oxygenation. Digits that have at least 95% saturation are well perfused, but values less than or equal to 84% require operative vascular treatment.[10]

Mangled upper extremities can still develop compartment syndrome despite the open wounds and a high index of suspicion needs to be maintained. Visually inspect and palpate for deformities, crepitus and tenderness to identify skeletal injuries. Asking the patient to move the digits and wrist can grossly assess the integrity of muscle-tendon units. Finally, examine the peripheral nerves including the median, radial, and ulnar. Not infrequently though, a definitive evaluation may need to be supplemented in the operating room.

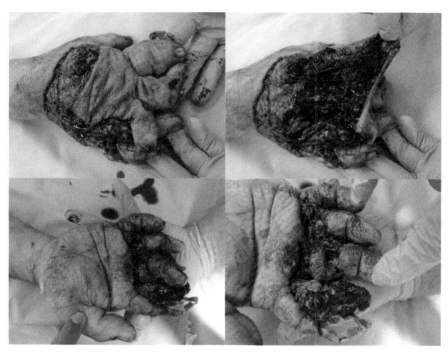

Fig. 1. Mangled hand injuries can be distracting due to their large wounds, gross deformities, and severe contamination.

Surgical Planning

Preoperatively, it is helpful to develop a surgical plan with some anticipation of potential donor sites for reconstruction. Otherwise, the surgeon may be frustrated by wasting valuable surgical time preparing additional sites for donor tissues. This may include the skin (thigh), vein (saphenous vein), or nerve (saphenous nerve).[3] For procedures involving amputated parts, having a backtable can be invaluable to begin identifying and tagging injured structures, shortening bone, and preparing for bony fixation.[6]

In general, the operation begins with an assessment of damaged structures and debridement. When a decision has been made to salvage the extremity, a suggested order of repair is bone, flexor tendons, extensor tendons, vein, artery, and nerve. If the injury is proximal and the distal limb is dysvascular, a vascular shunt should be considered, especially if extensive bony fixation is planned. It has been shown that revascularization should proceed before bony fixation in combined injuries to reduce morbidity.[11] Surgeons should also consider the use of spare parts for donor tissue, in which a nonreconstructable digit or structure is used for nerve, artery, vein, tendon, bone, or skin.

Operative Management

One of the first steps in the surgical management of mangled upper extremities is debridement.

Removing contamination and devitalized tissue prepares the wound for reconstruction, minimizes infection, and reduces the risks of systemic complications. Initial debridement can be done with the tourniquet inflated to aid in identifying and preserving critical structures. A methodical debridement of devitalized skin, muscle, tendon, and bone should be completed to create healthy surgical margins while preserving nerve and vascular structures. A temptation to retain marginal tissue should be avoided to ideally allow for early (<72 hrs) reconstruction. The wounds should then be irrigated.

Intraoperative cultures are typically not obtained. If a wound is heavily contaminated, a return debridement within 24 hours is indicated. During this debridement phase, the surgeon is also simultaneously assessing the damaged structures to determine if the limb is reconstructable. If so, the reconstruction typically begins with bony fixation.

Skeletal fixation

While the exact method of bony fixation depends on the trauma and is beyond the scope of this article, there are important guiding principles. The goals are to restore length, alignment, and stability, typically at the initial operation with the exception of severe contamination.[1] Obtaining stable fixation to allow early motion is especially critical in mangling upper extremity injuries because the tissues rapidly develop scar. Acute

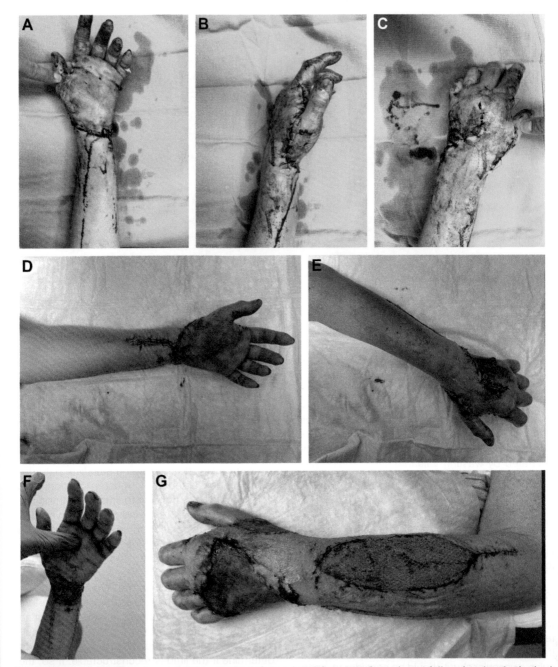

Fig. 2. The patient suffered a crush injury to the left hand and forearm after a horse fell on her (*A–C*). She had open distal radius and ulna fractures that were stabilized acutely after a thorough irrigation and debridement. There were also skin avulsion injuries to the palm and dorsal aspects of the hand. These are best managed by laying them back down rather than stretching the skin to close wounds. Otherwise, the marginal tissue can necrose (*D*). 24-hour after index surgery, patient developed compartment syndrome requiring release (*E*). Fortunately, larger areas of skin necrosis did not evolve and the wounds were ultimately managed with split-thickness skin grafts (*F, G*).

bone shortening can be considered to assist with managing bony defects and associated nerve and vessel injuries. About 1 to 1.5 cm of shortening can be tolerated in the phalanges and metacarpals, and up to 4 cm in the forearm.[1] Intra-articular fractures should be preserved unless a substantial portion is missing and would result in bone-to-bone contact. Primary bone

Defect Location	Defect Size	Treatment Choice
From fingertip to PIPJ 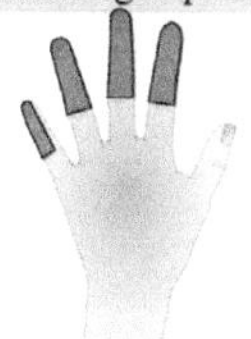	Small	Primary closure, Conventional local flap DAP flap
	Medium	DAP flap Reverse cross-finger flap (Younger) Artificial dermis with skin graft (Elder)
	Large	Distant flap (eg, Pedicle thin abdominal flap)
From PIPJ to MCPJ 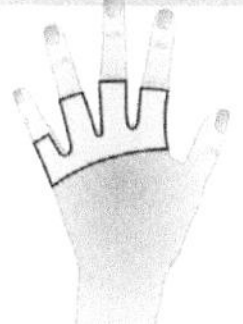	Small	Primary closure, Conventional local flap DMAP flap Flag flap, Axial flag flap, Reverse cross-finger flap
	Medium to Large	Retrograde flow flap (eg, Radial forearm flap, PIA flap) Free flap (eg, Dorsalis pedis flap, ALT flap) Distant flap (eg, Pedicle thin abdominal flap)
From MCPJ to Wrist 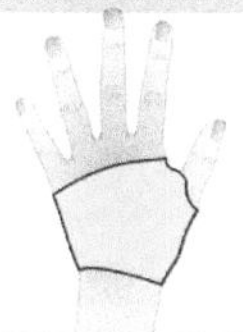	Small	Primary closure, Conventional local flap
	Medium	RAP flap (radial side), UAP flap (ulnar side) PIA flap
	Large	Free flap (eg, Dorsalis pedis flap, ALT flap) Distant flap (eg, Pedicle thin abdominal flap)
Dorsal thumb 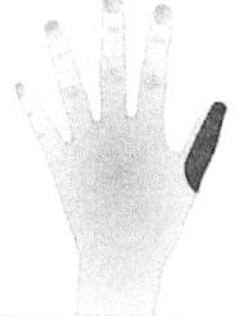	Small	Primary closure, Conventional local flap Reverse homodigital dorsoradial/dorsoulnar flaps
	Medium	FDMA flap
	Large	Free flap (eg, Dorsalis pedis flap) RAP flap, PIA flap

Fig. 3. Preferred flap options for dorsal hand defects. (Previously published materials unchanged from the source."From Ono S, Sebastin SJ, Ohi H, Chung KC. Microsurgical Flaps in Repair and Reconstruction of the Hand. Hand Clin 2017;33(3):425–41 https://doi.org/10.1016/j.hcl.2017.04.001. ; with permission")

grafting can be done to manage segmental bone defects as long as adequate debridement and soft tissue coverage can be obtained.[12] Alternatively, cement with or without antibiotics can be used as provisional spacers and later bone grafted after wound stabilization.[13] Larger defects (>6 cm) may require free vascularized bone flaps or vascularized bone transport.[6] While internal fixation and Kirschner wires are most commonly used for bony fixation, external fixators can provide skeletal stabilization when permanent hardware may be exposed with associated soft tissue injuries or infected by severe contamination.

Tendon repair
Tendon repairs are the next step. Unless ongoing limb ischemia is a concern, performing tendon repairs prior to nerve and vessels may decrease the chances of disrupting the microsurgical reconstruction. Standard techniques for primary tendon repairs are completed unless significant shortening or extreme joint positioning are needed. It not uncommon that the tendon ends are frayed and have loss tissue. Repairs may be facilitated by

bony shortening in these situations. Reconstruction is also an option with acute tendon grafting or staged using Silastic spacers. Proximal to flexor tendon zone 2 or extensor tendon zone 5, a tenodesis or tendon transfer can restore function, such as a side-to-side tenodesis of extensor tendons, or a sublimis to profundus transfer.[1]

Vascular repair/reconstruction
The success of vascular repair rests on careful microsurgical anastomosis and preparation of the vessel ends. An error is repairing an injured vessel on either side of the anastomosis.[1] Therefore, they need to be trimmed back until uninjured, healthy intima is seen. The resulting gap can be managed by bone shortening, flexing a joint, or a reversed vein graft. Options for vein graft material include the dorsal or volar forearm (for hand/fingers), dorsum of the foot (for hand/fingers), and the saphenous or cephalic veins (for brachial, radial, and ulnar artery). A pitfall during vein grafting is using too long of a graft, predisposing it to kinking and thrombosis.[1] Predilating the vein graft after reversal using 10 U/mL of heparinized saline

Defect Location	Defect Size	Treatment Choice
● From fingertip to PIPJ	Small	Secondary intension (if bone is not exposed)
		V-Y advancement flap, Oblique triangular flap
		Thenar flap (Younger), Homodigital island flap
		Toe pulp free flap
	Medium to Large	Heterodigital island flap
		Free flap (SPBRA flap, Mediais pedis flap)
● From PIPJ to MCPJ	Small	Primary closure, Conventional local flap
		Heterodigital island flap
	Medium	Free flap (SPBRA flap, Medialis pedis flap)
		Axial flag flap, Cross-finger flap
	Large	Free flap (eg, Medialis pedis flap, ALT flap)
		Distant flap (eg, Pedicle thin abdominal flap)
● From MCPJ to Wrist	Small	Conventional local flap
		Secondary intension (if vital structures are not exposed)
	Medium-to-Large	Free medialis pedis flap
		Free flap (eg, ALT flap)
		Distant flap (eg, Pedicle thin abdominal flap)
● Palmar thumb 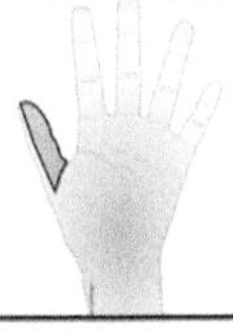	Small	Moberg advancement flap
	Medium	Heterodigital island flap
		Toe pulp free flap
	Large	Free medialis pedis flap
		Distant flap (eg, Pedicle thin abdominal flap)

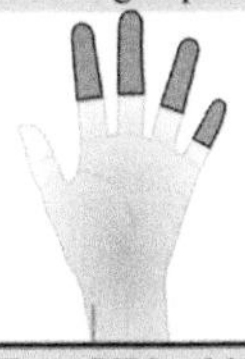

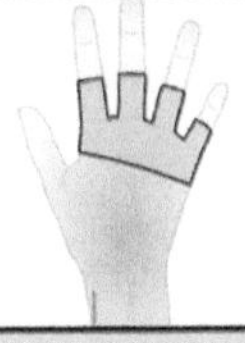

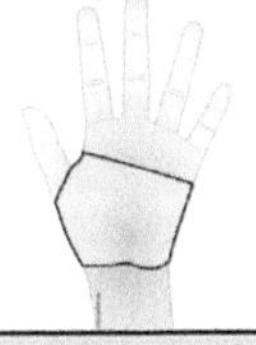

Fig. 4. Preferred flap options for palmar hand defects. (Previously published materials unchanged from the source:"From Ono S, Sebastin SJ, Ohi H, Chung KC. Microsurgical Flaps in Repair and Reconstruction of the Hand. Hand Clin 2017;33(3):425–41 https://doi.org/10.1016/j.hcl.2017.04.001. ; with permission")

can assist with measuring the correct length of graft prior to distal anastomosis. Intra-venous heparin administration during digital replants or revascularizations have not been shown to have a clear positive impact on success.[14]

Nerve repair/reconstruction

Nerves are usually managed toward the end of the case after vascular reconstruction. If the nerve is in continuity, it can be left alone and function monitored postoperatively for spontaneous recovery. If a nerve is lacerated or avulsed, we advocate performing an acute nerve repair or reconstruction. An argument could be made to delay nerve grafting until a secondary procedure is performed in case the wound is contaminated and infection causes the loss of graft material.[1] A tension-less, primary nerve repair after trimming the ends back to healthy fascicles is ideal. If this cannot be achieved, typically an autograft or allograft nerve is needed. There is a growing body of literature supporting equivalent rates of meaningful sensory and motor recovery using allo-versus autograft nerves.[15]

Soft tissue coverage

The ideal healed wound is stable, durable, and vascularized. Soft tissue coverage is evaluated at the time of the initial surgery. It is preferable to obtain early soft tissue coverage (<72 hours) to reduce infection, wound and bone healing complications, and the length of hospital stay.[16] In the senior author's opinion, a definitive closure or soft tissue reconstruction can be completed acutely if the wound is not severely contaminated. Otherwise, a thorough debridement to convert the wound into clean-contaminated, and repeat a serial debridement in 24 to 48 hours. If possible, a soft tissue reconstruction is performed then. Temporary coverage with Integra or negative-pressure wound device can be a good option in the intervening period.

The concept of the reconstructive ladder is well described. In the upper extremity, choosing the simplest option that achieves optimal form and function is preferred over simply choosing the simplest option.[1] The size of the wound and the presence of "white" structures (tendon, nerve, vessel, bone, ligament/joint) often dictate the sof tissue coverage. Whenever possible, primary closure should be performed. In the case of traumatically elevated skin flaps, the surgeon should lay down the skin rather than stretch it back to its original position.[1] Doing so may limit further ischemia of marginal tissue. Smaller resulting wounds can be left to heal by secondary intention. This scenario may be better than a large wound dehiscence or subsequent necrosis of a large area of the skin flap. Other times, a skin graft may be fine except over exposed bone without periosteum or tendon without paratenon (**Fig. 2**).

A variety of local, regional, and free flaps are available. Selecting the right flap is challenging. Multiple factors can affect the choice including the size and location of the wound, flap characteristics, patient characteristics and preferences, and surgeon knowledge and experience. In the hand, the senior author has presented his preferences for soft tissue coverage (**Figs. 3** and **4**).[17] When deciding on a flap for the hand, the surgeon should consider size, location, and tissue characteristics. In general, smaller defects can be closed primarily or with conventional local flaps. Medium-sized defects are preferentially reconstructed with perforator flaps, especially propellor designs.[18]

Advantages of a perforator flap include being thin, pliable, improved aesthetic outcomes because of like-with-like reconstruction, and minimal donor site morbidity by leaving muscle in-situ.

Whenever possible, reconstructing like with like tissue provides improved functional and aesthetic outcomes.[17] Additionally, the dorsal and palmar aspects of the hand are functionally different. The palmar skin is thicker, hair-less and resistant to shearing through its attachments to the palmar aponeurosis. In contrast, the dorsal skin is thinner and more mobile to accommodate to joint flexion and extension. A dorsal flap is preferentially used for dorsal defects, and a palmar flap for the palmar surface. Large defects generally require free or distal flaps. There are more choices available for large dorsal hand defects, but the foot remains the only source of glabrous skin.[17] The medialis pedis flap is a good option for palmar defects, but typically limited to a defect size of 5 × 10 cm.[17]

Flaps are also typically needed in large forearm wounds or with exposed "white" structures. However, consider closing smaller wounds or skin grafting whenever possible. Around the elbow, flaps are usually needed as well because underlying "white" structures or prostheses/hardware are

Table 1
Flap options around the elbow and forearm

	Destination	Advantages
Fasciocutaneous		
Radial forearm	Small- or medium-sized defects around posterior elbow, antecubital fossa, or proximal forearm	• Long pedicle • Pliable soft tissue • Ease of dissection
Reverse lateral arm flap	Small- or medium-sized defects around lateral or posterior elbow	• Avoids sacrificing major upper extremity artery
Anterolateral thigh flap	Broad application for coverage of large- to massive defects around elbow/forearm	• Versatile • Easier flap elevation for secondary procedures than muscle flaps
Muscle		
Flexor carpi ulnaris or brachioradialis	Small- or medium-sized defects around the elbow	• Minimal donor site morbidity
Latissimus dorsi	Broad application for coverage of large- to massive defects around elbow/forearm	• Versatile, reliable with large available dimensions up to 25 × 35 cm • Muscle effectively fills dead spaces
Distant flaps		
Thoraco-abdominal pedicled flaps	Larger wounds in the forearm	• Useful when other options are inappropriate or unavailable

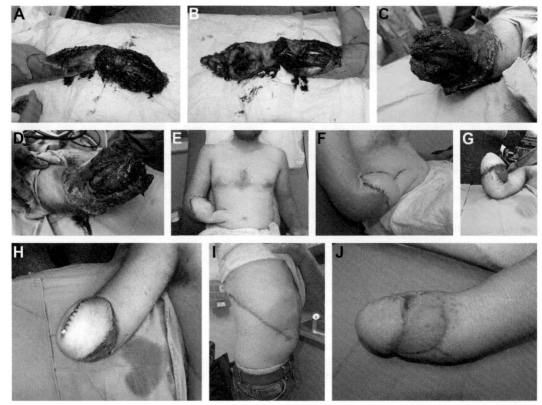

Fig. 5. The patient suffered a severe crush avulsion injury to right forearm (*A, B*). This was managed with debridement and acute amputation (*C, D*). The wound was reconstructed in 24 hours using a 31 × 10 cm thoracoabdominal pedicle flap based on the rectus perforator (*E, F*). The brachioradialis was divided into thirds and used to wrap around the ulnar, median, and radial nerves for the future nerve interface coverage. At 3 weeks, the flap was divided (*G, H*) and final wound appearance (*I, J*).

easily exposed. Various distant, pedicled, and free flap choices are available, each with their advantages and uses (**Table 1**) (**Fig. 5**).[19]

SUMMARY

In conclusion, mutilating upper extremity injuries are complex requiring an understanding of multiple disciplines including orthopedics, plastic surgery, and vascular. Initial management entails preserving life over limb, but reconstructive surgery of the mangled upper extremity aims to preserve function. General principles of surgical management are "radical," aggressive initial debridement of devitalized tissue, and converting the contaminated wound to a clean-contaminated one. Additionally, the surgeon should aim for rigid skeletal stabilization to allow early joint motion whereby possible. Healing and functional recovery are also highly dependent on achieving a stable, vascularized soft tissue coverage. We emphasize obtaining definitive wound management early (<72 hours).

CLINICS CARE POINTS

- Remember life over limb always.
- Aggressive initial debridement and conversion of wound to a clean-contaminated one.
- Tissue scarring develops early. Obtaining stable bony fixation to allow early joint motion is one of the only ways to mitigate against otherwise inevitable stiffness and contracture.
- Early (<72 hours), definitive soft tissue coverage reduces infection, promotes bone healing, lessens the length of hospital stay, and ultimately optimizes outcomes.

DISCLOSURE

T.K.K. Chan has no disclosure. Dr K.C. Chung receives funding from the National Institutes of Health, United States and book royalties from Wolters Kluwer and Elsevier.

REFERENCES

1. Green DP, Wolfe SW. Green's operative hand surgery. Philadelphia, PA: Elsevier/Churchill Livingstone; 2011.
2. Moran SL, Berger RA. Biomechanics and hand trauma: what you need. Hand Clin 2003;19(1):17–31.
3. Lahiri A. Managing mutilating hand injuries. Clin Plast Surg 2019;46(3):351–7.
4. Soucacos PN. Indications and selection for digital amputation and replantation. J Hand Surg Br 2001;26(6):572–81.
5. Peacock EE, Van Winkle W. Surgery and biology of wound repair. Philadelphia, PA: W.B. Saunders; 1970.
6. Tosti R, Eberlin KR. "Damage control" hand surgery: evaluation and emergency management of the mangled hand. Hand Clin 2018;34(1):17–26.
7. Pederson WC. Replantation. Plast Reconstr Surg 2001;107(3):823–41.
8. VanderWilde RS, Wood MB, Zu ZG. Hand replantation after 54 hours of cold ischemia: a case report. J Hand Surg Am 1992;17(2):217–20.
9. Wei FC, Chang YL, Chen HC, et al. Three successful digital replantations in a patient after 84, 86, and 94 hours of cold ischemia time. Plast Reconstr Surg 1988;82(2):346–50.
10. Tarabadkar N, Iorio ML, Gundle K, et al. The use of pulse oximetry for objective quantification of vascular injuries in the hand. Plast Reconstr Surg 2015;136(6):1227–33.
11. McHenry TP, Holcomb JB, Aoki N, et al. Fractures with major vascular injuries from gunshot wounds: implications of surgical sequence. J Trauma 2002;53(4):717–21.
12. Saint-Cyr M, Gupta A. Primary internal fixation and bone grafting for open fractures of the hand. Hand Clin 2006;22(3):317–27.
13. Masquelet AC. Induced membrane technique: pearls and pitfalls. J Orthop Trauma 2017;31(Suppl 5):S36–8.
14. Deblois S, Zhu L, Mastropasqua B, et al. The clinical effectiveness and safety of intravenous unfractionated heparin following digital replantation and revascularization: a narrative systematic review. Microsurgery 2022;42(6):622–30.
15. Lans J, Eberlin KR, Evans PJ, et al. A systematic review and meta-analysis of nerve gap repair: comparative effectiveness of allografts, autografts, and conduits. Plast Reconstr Surg 2023;151(5):814e–27e.
16. Godina M. Early microsurgical reconstruction of complex trauma of the extremities. Plast Reconstr Surg 1986;78(3):285–92.
17. Ono S, Sebastin SJ, Ohi H, et al. Microsurgical flaps in repair and reconstruction of the hand. Hand Clin 2017;33(3):425–41.
18. Ono S, Sebastin SJ, Yazaki N, et al. Clinical applications of perforator-based propeller flaps in upper limb soft tissue reconstruction. J Hand Surg Am 2011;36(5):853–63.
19. Adkinson JM, Chung KC. Flap reconstruction of the elbow and forearm: a case-based approach. Hand Clin 2014;30(2):153–63.

Free Functional Muscle Transfer—Technical Considerations

Utkan Aydin, MD[a],*, Kevin C. Chung, MD, MS[b]

KEYWORDS

- Free muscle transfer • Upper extremity • Ischemic contracture • Tendons

KEY POINTS

- Free functional muscle transfer combines techniques and principles used for both microsurgery and tendon transfers.
- Restoration of finger and restoration of elbow flexion are the most common applications of free functional muscle transfers in the upper extremity.
- After over 50 years in the reconstructive armamentarium of the upper extremity surgeons, it has evolved into a safe procedure with good functional outcomes.

INTRODUCTION

Free functional muscles were first used to improve function in the upper extremity over 50 years ago.[1] Up until then, only palliative surgical interventions such as arthrodesis, osteotomies, and even amputations were considered as treatment options in cases with extensive loss of functioning muscles in the extremities. This procedure enabled the replacement of a missing muscle-tendon unit and its function and is often regarded as the best option where there are no expendable tendons or muscles for transfer locally.

This sophisticated procedure necessitates excellence in diverse domains of hand surgery. It is a combination of a free tissue transfer, which requires meticulous microsurgical technique, and a tendon transfer which in turn requires a thorough understanding of tendon biomechanics and familiarity with a wide range of postoperative therapy modalities.

In many cases, free functional muscle transfer (FFMT) is the only available reconstructive option to restore loss of motion. Extensive loss of the muscle-tendon unit is the most common indication for FFMT, with Volkmann ischemic contracture being the typical candidate for this procedure. Besides, patients who lost function because of trauma (burns, infections), oncologic resection, nerve damage, extensive brachial plexus injuries, and even congenital malformations can benefit from FFMTs.[2–6]

Brief history of the procedure

The first report of successful free muscle transfer in an experimental canine model was made by Tamai and colleagues in 1970.[1] The investigators provided electrophysiologic and electron microscopic evidence that the transferred rectus femoris muscle recovered functionality 3 months after neurovascular coaptations. The clinical use of

---

[a] Hand Surgery Section, Department of Orthopedic Surgery and Hand Surgery, Akademiska Hospital, Uppsala 751 85, Sweden; [b] Department of Surgery, Section of Plastic Surgery, University of Michigan Medical School, Ann Arbor, MI, USA
* Corresponding author. Hand Surgery Section, Department of Orthopedic Surgery and Hand Surgery, Akademiska Hospital, Uppsala 751 85, Sweden.
E-mail address: utkana@hotmail.com

Clin Plastic Surg 51 (2024) 505–514
https://doi.org/10.1016/j.cps.2024.02.016

FFMTs was reported a couple of years later by various research teams for facial and upper extremity reanimation.[7,8]

EVALUATION

FFMT is the microsurgical transfer of a muscle which can contract voluntarily to provide active motion to tendons with non-functioning muscle-tendon units. Therefore, many aspects of preoperative patient evaluation bear similarities to tendon transfers and free flap surgery.

Because the active range of motion (ROM) after the FFMT cannot exceed the passive ROM of the joints involved, the prerequisite of a successful FFMT is supple joints. Passive ROM of the joints should be maximized preoperatively, and improvements to passive ROM achieved after rehabilitation should be deemed as sustainable in the long term. Achieving this will even require staged interventions such as arthrolysis, tenolysis, and contracture releases.

Most patients who undergo FFMTs have previously sustained extensive muscle loss, meaning that the active motion of several joints located in the same line of motion might be absent, such as finger and wrist flexors in case of muscle loss in the forearm. The use of a single muscle unit which can voluntarily contract leads to a compound motion, like the simultaneous flexion of the fingers and wrist. This might seem to contradict with the tendon transfers principle called "1 muscle, 1 function" and is unfortunately an unavoidable consequence of the scarcity of functioning muscle-tendon units. Therefore, the surgeon should predict the resulting motion after an FFMT and plan countermeasures to optimize it. Arthrodesis of the wrist may be required to improve grasp function; otherwise, tenodesis of the finger extensors may be necessary. Most importantly, any skeletal instability should be addressed before surgery for FFMT.

There is also a need for a counteracting force to balance the pull of the transferred muscle. The absence of such will lead to an extremity stuck at total flexion or extension. The counteracting muscle should be strong enough to overcome the pull of the transferred muscle to ensure an acceptable amount of motion within a functional range. When both flexor and extensor function in the hand and fingers need to be reconstructed, the treatment has to be staged, and FFMT for extension function should be done before the restoration of flexion to facilitate postoperative rehabilitation.

FFMT enables simultaneous transfer of skin and fascia in addition to functional muscle. Thus, areas with extensive scarring or tight soft tissue coverage can be reconstructed in a single session. Both donor muscles frequently used for FFMT, gracilis and latissimus dorsi, can be raised with a reliable skin paddle to add skin to the recipient area if it is needed.

To ensure the presence of viable recipient vessels, especially in the extremities which sustained extensive soft tissue trauma, the use of various vascular imaging techniques should be considered. Before the harvest of the functional muscle, Doppler investigation of the skin paddle overlying the muscle will help to identify perforating vessels from the muscle and hence increase the reliability of the transferred skin and fascia.

Another crucial factor to consider prior to any attempt to use FFMT is to ensure that the candidate for this procedure is well informed, ready, and motivated enough to begin a long and sometimes quite arduous journey. Establishing realistic expectations, a readiness to deal with complications, and the long rehabilitation period after surgery renders a patient more compliant, leading to better outcomes for the patient. The patient should also be made aware of the timeframe for when the expected result after an FFMT will be apparent, which in most cases will take a year or more.

Diminished regeneration potential due to advanced age and or increased load on the transferred muscle because of obesity can lead to inferior results. Patients with comorbidities that can complicate a long microvascular procedure and a prolonged rehabilitation process are not ideal candidates for this procedure.

APPROACH

The most common indications for FFMT are the loss of forearm muscles in cases with Volkmann ischemic contracture and the loss of elbow flexors. Other indications follow the same approach except for brachial plexus injuries which will often require a modified treatment algorithm, especially regarding the selection and preparation of recipient nerves.

A thorough history detailing the medical condition of the patient and the injury mechanism is needed to exclude unsuitable patients. Radiographs of the involved extremity are necessary to rule out skeletal deformities. It must be kept in mind that patients who experience reduced sensation in their hands or have poor eyesight are unsuitable candidates because of the loss of proprioception to use the reconstructed limb.

Videos are an indispensable tool to document the function in the extremity preoperatively. The British Medical Council (BMC) Scale is widely used to measure muscle strength. Patient-reported outcome measures such as the Michigan Hand Outcomes Questionnaire and the Shortened Disabilities of the Arm, Shoulder, and Hand Questionnaire are also helpful to document the global extremity function from the patient's perspective before surgery.[9] Chronic pain conditions, especially those affecting the involved extremity, should be addressed preoperatively along with the possible effects of FFMT on these conditions. The expectations of the patient must also be discussed.

Preoperative electrophysiologic tests will help to get a detailed picture of the status of the nerves. The presence of activity in the pronator muscle suggests an intact anterior interosseous nerve (AIN), which is an ideal nerve recipient nerve for a functional muscle to reconstruct finger flexion.

Initiation of intensive rehabilitation regiments should be considered in patients if there seems to be any potential to improve mobility as well as preventive measures, such as splints, to avoid deformities.

An ideal muscle for FFMT should be expendable and not lead to any functional deficit when harvested, have a consistent vascular anatomy and enough pedicle length, and enough excursion to provide the desired amount of motion. Preferably, the resulting scar from the harvest should not be immediately visible and the muscle's location should permit a 2-team approach to shorten the duration of the surgical procedure. Taking all these points into consideration, gracilis and latissimus dorsi muscles appear to be the 2 best options for FFMTs.

Harvest of gracilis muscle

The recipient site on the upper extremity is usually prepared first before the harvest of the muscle to make sure that there are suitable recipient nerve or nerves to connect to the motor nerve of the gracilis muscle and the vessels are ready for anastomosis.

The gracilis muscle is a thigh adductor and is located on the medial aspect of the thigh. It takes its origin off ischiopubic ramus and the tendon of the muscle inserts to medial condyle on the tibia. The width of the muscle is 5 to 8 cm, and its length is 20 to 30 cm in adults, although its dimensions vary with body composition. The thickness of gracilis is 2 to 3 cm on average. The tendinous part of the muscle on its distal end is around 15 cm and is even longer in some cases.

The blood supply of the gracilis muscle follows type II pedicle pattern according to Mathes and Nahai classification and has a minor vascular

pedicle in addition to a dominant pedicle, although some variation may exist in the pedicle anatomy. The dominant vascular pedicle arises from the medial femoral circumflex artery which is a branch of the deep femoral artery and enters the muscle on its posteromedial surface (**Fig. 1**). The dominant pedicle is usually located 6 to 12 cm distal to the pubic tubercle. In addition, branches arising directly from the deep femoral artery constitute minor vascular pedicles. To gain more pedicle length and increase the diameter of the anastomosis, the vessels should be dissected free proximally up to the level of the deep femoral artery. The diameter of the arterial pedicle is 1.5 mm on average and the accompanying vein has an average diameter of 2.0 mm. Venae comitantes join to form a large but short vein which drains into the deep femoral vein. The saphenous vein is also located in the flap territory and can be included during harvest and might function as a backup vein for the skin paddle.

Because most of the musculocutaneous perforators are in the proximal one-third of the flap, a more reliable skin paddle can be prepared based on those; however, the skin paddle is still prone to necrosis especially in patients with increased subcutaneous fat. The sensory innervation of the flap territory is provided by medial cutaneous nerve of the thigh.

Although the entire muscle is innervated by the anterior branch of the obturator nerve, it can be dissected in fascicles to use the muscle for 2 separate functions by connecting these to 2 different recipient nerves. Use of a nerve stimulator can facilitate identification of the muscle territories innervated by individual fascicles. The nerve enters the muscle a couple of centimeters more proximal than the vascular pedicle.

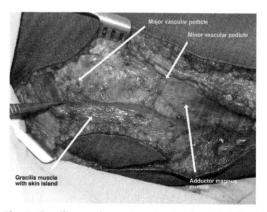

Fig. 1. Gracilis muscle can be raised with a skin island. The major vascular pedicle arises from the medial femoral circumflex artery. Minor pedicles usually arise from the superficial femoral artery.

Gracilis lies over the adductor longus and is located distally between the sartorius and semitendinosus muscles. The common insertion of the sartorius, semitendinosus, and the gracilis muscles on anteromedial aspect of the tibia is called "pes anserinus" and additional tendon length can be gained by harvesting the periosteum in this area if needed. This might require 2 separate incisions to avoid a long single scar on the medial thigh (Fig. 2).

Preoperative marking of the course of gracilis facilitates its harvest. The first step is to identify the adductor longus muscle on the medial thigh. Both adductor longus and gracilis muscles become prominent when the hip is flexed, adducted, and externally rotated (frog-leg position). Gracilis and adductor longus muscles form a groove in the proximal medial thigh, which can be palpated in muscular individuals. The course of gracilis follows a line 2 to 3 cm inferior to a line drawn between medial femoral condyle and adductor insertion to the pubis.

The easiest patient position for flap harvest is the frog-leg position with the hip flexed, externally rotated, and adducted. Adductor longus muscle is easily confused with gracilis, which lies posterior to the former. After incision of skin and fascia, the junction between adductor longus and gracilis is identified and retracting adductor longus anteriorly

exposes the vascular pedicle. Following dissection of the pedicle, the tendon of the muscle is transected, and the flap is raised in a distal to proximal direction by freeing it from adductor longus anteriorly and adductor magnus posteriorly. Gracilis can be harvested with adductor longus because they share the same vascular pedicle and motor innervation.

The fascia surrounding the muscle should be left intact because this will improve muscle gliding of the distal tendon. Before releasing the resting tension of the muscle by transection of its insertion or its origin, several sutures should be placed in regular intervals and the tension of the muscle after its transfer should be set to bring the sutures in this same distance from each other. This will reestablish optimal overlap of muscle filament and prevent over-tensioning or under-tensioning. Extension of the knee and abduction of the hip will bring the muscle to an adequate physiologically fully stretched length.

Several minor pedicles arising from deep femoral artery along the anterior surface of the adductor magnus should be ligated. The last step is the separation of the muscle from its proximal origin. Ischemia time will be kept at a minimum if the preparation of recipient area is completed before the division of the vascular pedicle. Following harvest, the skin is closed in layers and an active drain is placed. Pressure dressings can help to prevent seroma formation.

Preparation of the recipient area

Previous scars on the recipient area and the location of the potential donor nerves used to innervate the free muscle dictate how the exposure of the recipient area should be planned (Fig. 3). The planned exposure should allow excision of all fibrotic muscle as well.

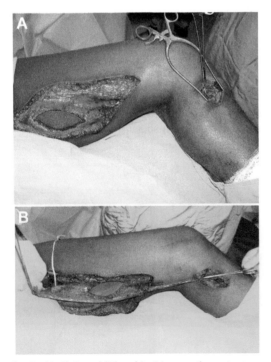

Fig. 2. (A, B) An additional incision on the anteromedial surface of the proximal tibia while lifting the gracilis flap makes the harvest of a longer tendinous portion possible.

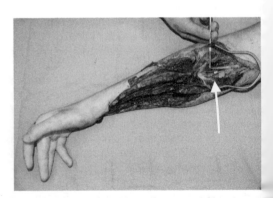

Fig. 3. Release and excision of scars and fibrotic muscle results in a large skin and soft tissue defect. One of the advantages of free functional gracilis muscle transfer is that it can simultaneously restore voluntary action and reconstruct large defects.

An ideal motor nerve to innervate the transferred muscle should lie outside of the zone of injury and preferably have a similar number of axons and a similar function aimed to reconstruct through FFMT to facilitate rehabilitation. In most cases with Volkmann contractures, the nerves previously innervating the absent muscles are available. Recipient nerves must be freed of neuromas, and the nerve fascicles must be exposed in the distal end of the nerve to make a functioning nerve coaptation. Frozen section of the nerve ends can help if there are any doubts about the presence of axons. Potential recipient nerves should be stimulated to confirm their functionality by observing contractions if there are still muscle remnants left attached to them.

The presence of flow in arteries adjacent to nerves at angiography suggests intact nerves. This finding can be especially useful if the AIN is chosen as the motor recipient in the forearm.[10,11] If AIN is not available, branches of ulnar nerve are also good alternatives. AIN can be divided into its fascicles if the transferred muscle will be split to provide independent actions.

Placing the nerve coaptation as close to the muscle as possible will shorten the time needed for the reinnervation of the transferred muscle. Nerve grafts can be used but will result in worse outcomes compared with direct coaptation of donor and recipient nerves.

It should be kept in mind that the pedicle of the transferred muscle and hence the anastomosis will move with the contraction of the muscle. The geometry of the anastomosis should be planned accordingly, and the tension of the anastomosis should accommodate some mobility within the range of muscle excursion.

The ulnar artery, radial artery, or anterior interosseous artery can be chosen for microvascular anastomosis in the forearm. Depending on the vascularization pattern in the involved extremity, which might have changed because of trauma or prior surgery, end-to-side coaptation might be an alternative. The superficial veins of the upper extremity are more prone to trauma, and their diameter might not match with concomitant veins of the transferred muscle rendering the venae comitantes of the forearm arteries as a better choice for vein anastomosis. In the case of gracilis muscle transfer, if the saphenous vein was included in the flap, this can be anastomosed to the superficial veins of the upper extremity.

Reconstruction of finger flexion

The medial epicondyle, which is the origin of the native flexor muscles of the forearm, is used to attach the transferred muscle for finger flexion. The existing skin envelope in the forearm may not be sufficient to accommodate increased volume coming from the transferred muscle. If that is the case, a large skin island must be raised attached to the functional muscle, this is possible for both latissimus dorsi and gracilis muscles.

To avoid postoperative flexion contracture from over-tensioning or lack flexion power from under-tensioning, the tension is adjusted with the hand and fingers in full extension and then the muscle is stretched to its resting length by bringing the suture markings on the muscle to the same intervals before harvest.[12] The level of distal tendon repair between the deep finger flexors and the tendon of the transferred muscle is then marked in this position. The wrist should be brought to flexion again during tendon repair to make a repair without tension. Pulvertaft weave or side-to-side tendon repair techniques can be used. To prevent adhesions, superficial finger flexors should be excised. The cascade of the fingers, with incrementally increasing flexion from index to little finger should be reestablished and can be done by bundling and suturing them together at the right tension while keeping them in their correct positions according to the cascade (**Figs. 4 and 5**).

When doing the distal tendon repair, the tension of the flexor pollicis longus should be adjusted in a way permitting it to flex slightly less than the fingers to prevent the thumb from ending up in the palm during the compound grasp motion. If the simultaneous flexion of thumb and fingers with the contraction of the transferred muscle is not desired, the muscle should be divided into 2 functional units by dissecting the motor nerve and separating fascicles to innervate distinct parts of the muscle. Two separate healthy recipient nerves must be available for independent stimulation and contraction of those distinct parts.

Reconstruction of elbow flexion

To reconstruct elbow flexion, the origin of the transferred muscle is fixed to the lateral one-third of the clavicle and acromion (**Figs. 6–8**). If available, the biceps tendon is the best option for distal tendon repair; in its absence, the tendon can be anchored to the radius or ulna.

The spinal accessory nerve should be the first choice for nerve coaptation. Intercostal nerves have been used with acceptable results as recipient nerves, especially in cases with brachial plexus injuries (**Figs. 9 and 10**).

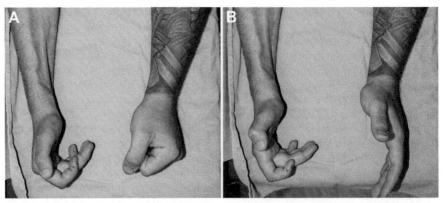

Fig. 4. (*A*) The patient was asked to make a fist. He presented with a loss of active flexion of the fingers of the right hand after extensive injury of the flexor muscles in the volar forearm. (*B*) Same patient while he attempts to extend his fingers. Fibrosis in the volar forearm led to a flexion contracture of the fingers.

Postoperative care

The early postoperative period requires close meticulous monitoring of the free flap to avoid failure. Muscle tissue is more intolerant to ischemia compared to many other tissues such as the skin or fascia. Additionally, prolonged periods of ischemia will lead to complete failure or suboptimal results. The manifestation of clinical signs of flap failure will be delayed on the skin paddle, so

it is advised to add more advanced modalities of flap monitorization such as an invasive/noninvasive Doppler.

The elbow is splinted at 90° in flexion postoperatively if an FFMT is done for elbow flexion until the patient felt spontaneous muscle contraction. Once this happens, continued electric stimulation of the muscle to promote hypertrophy is useful. The patient is kept splinted with the elbow at 90° of flexion to prevent muscle stretching. Once the

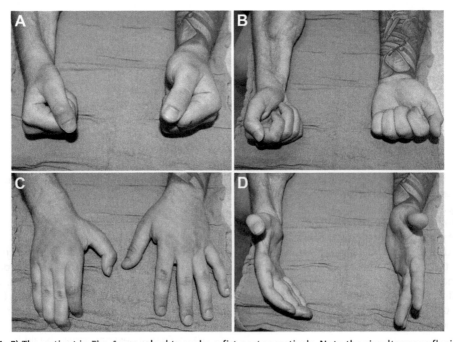

Fig. 5. (*A, B*) The patient in **Fig. 4** was asked to make a fist postoperatively. Note the simultaneous flexion of the thumb in the operated right hand. (*C, D*) In addition to restoring active flexion, an increase of active extension is seen postoperatively resulting from the release of scars and fibrotic muscles. The patient has regained his ability to grasp which leads to a significant improvement of the patient's extremity function while conducting daily activities.

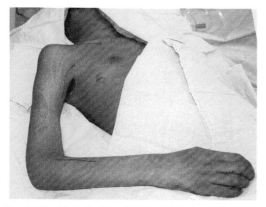

Fig. 6. Markings before free functional muscle transfer (FFMT) using a gracilis free flap for the restoration of elbow flexion. The areas marked are the clavicle, axilla, and the proximal forearm.

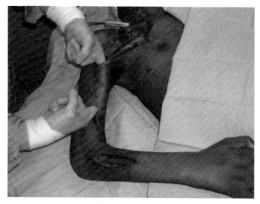

Fig. 8. Creating a subcutaneous tunnel by connecting the clavicular and upper arm incisions allows a flap inset with shorter incisions.

patient has sufficient strength to keep the muscle at 30° of flexion, the splint can cease, and patient is encouraged to move the elbow as much as possible to conduct daily activities. Results will often not be optimal until after 2 years.

CLINICAL OUTCOMES

Almost 50 years have passed since the first report of an FFMT. Today, the technique has been refined, and the outcomes of the procedure show that it can be performed safely and with reproducible, satisfactory results (see **Figs. 4, 5** and **10**).

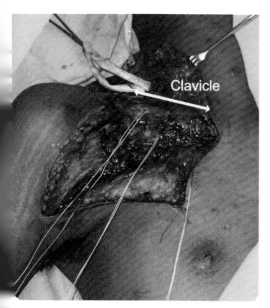

Fig. 7. Preparation of the clavicle for the insertion of the gracilis muscle for the restoration of elbow flexion.

There is no consensus in the literature on how to define a successful outcome after an FFMT. Grip and pinch strength are commonly used after the restoration of finger flexion as well as ROM and muscle strength according to the BMC Scale.

As with any microsurgical procedure, perioperative and early postoperative complications may arise. Common problems after long surgeries such as pressure wounds and pulmonary complications should be prevented using standard measures. Muscle herniation at the donor site can be a problem if the fascial layer is not closed properly.

In a review article, Zuker[10] reported that more than half of the patients who underwent FFMT to flexor forearm were able to make a complete fist. Another series with 22 Volkmann ischemic contracture patients reported that 20 of these patients who recovered M3/M4 motor power for finger flexion expressed high satisfaction with the operation.[13] In a more heterogenous case series including patients with obstetric and adult brachial plexus injuries as well as congenital upper

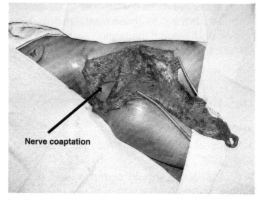

Fig. 9. Coaptation of the spinal accessory nerve to the obturator nerve of the gracilis muscle.

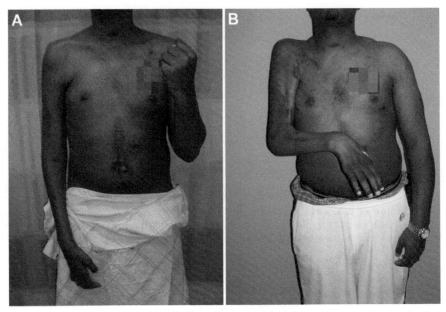

Fig. 10. (*A*) Preoperative patient with a loss of elbow flexion in his right upper extremity due to the absence of muscles in the upper arm. (*B*) Patient after the restoration of elbow flexion. The patient underwent a wrist arthrodesis in a later stage.

extremity conditions, the investigators stated that 70% of patients had successful outcomes.[14]

The most common indication for FFMT for elbow flexion is brachial plexus injuries. A systematic review comparing FFMTs and non–free-flap procedures for restoration of elbow flexion revealed that FFMTs resulted in higher mean strength scores and lower failure rates.[15] Non–free-flap procedures included in this review were muscle transfers such as pectoralis and latissimus dorsi transfer, the Steindler procedure, and nerve transfers such as the Oberlin procedure.

Secondary procedures are not uncommon; especially tenolysis and contracture releases addressing overtightened tendons may become necessary. Children who underwent FFMTs before growth spurs are more susceptible to developing deformities leading to those interventions. Night splinting until skeletal maturation can help to prevent deformities.[10,11] Moving the insertion of the

elbow flexor distally can improve active ROM in cases with suboptimal results after elbow flexion reconstruction with FFMT.[16]

FUTURE DIRECTIONS

There is promising progress regarding the creation of a skeletal muscle construct with bioengineering that will be implanted and become functional in the human body, although the research is still in its early stages.[17] Bioengineered muscles can be customized according to the specific needs of the patient and avoid donor site morbidity.

Endoscopic methods of harvest for both latissimus dorsi and gracilis muscles have been described.[18] However, the use of the flap as a functional muscle after harvest has not gained popularity yet. Refining endoscopic techniques

---

Box 1
Microsurgery

- Minimize ischemia.
- Nerve coaptation as close to muscle as possible.
- Pedicle length should permit muscle movement during contraction.
- Close monitorization.

Box 2
Tendon/muscle transfer

- Passive range of motion should be optimized preoperatively.
- Adequate soft tissue coverage around tendons/muscle-tendon junction is necessary to permit gliding.
- The tension of the muscle must be adjusted correctly.
- Physical/occupational therapy is a crucial component of treatment.

> **Box 3**
> **Reconstruction of finger flexion**
>
> - Suture finger flexors together to establish the right cascade.
> - The flexor pollicis longus should flex later than other fingers.
> - There should be an extending counterforce to balance flexion.

- Every effort should be made to maximally optimize the conditions in each step. Ensuring good passive ROM preoperatively, avoiding prolonged ischemia perioperatively, and intensive rehabilitation postoperatively will help to achieve better results.
- Studies have so far reported consistently good functional results after FFMTs. It will be a life-changing intervention for good candidates.

has the potential to reduce donor side morbidity and the duration of the surgery, but it comes with a learning curve until consistent results are achieved.

Another potential use of FFMTs is the restoration of elbow flexion in patients with arthrogryposis. There are case reports and small case series reporting the use of FFMT for this indication, but more research is needed before it can be recommended as a viable treatment option for this indication.[14,19,20]

There are reports of using both a segment of gracilis muscle and other muscles such as pronator quadratus, pectoralis major, serratus anterior, abductor hallucis, and extensor digitorum brevis as a free functional muscle to reconstruct defects in the thenar region. Despite good outcomes reported by the investigators, the number of cases who underwent these surgeries is currently limited and the superiority of these techniques compared with standard tendon transfers is still unclear.[21,22]

SUMMARY

The use of FFMT in the reconstruction of the upper extremity has proved to be a safe and reliable method with reproducible outcomes. Although the use of FFMTs was previously limited to a few medical centers, it is now available as a treatment to a much wider population. This has accelerated improvements in the surgical technique as well as postoperative rehabilitation protocols, and at the same time, assessment of outcomes has become more reliable because of larger case series. Adhering to the established principles mentioned in this article will facilitate achieving satisfactory and consistent results (**Box 1–3**).

CLINICS CARE POINTS

- Selection of clinically suitable and motivated patients for this procedure with a long rehabilitation period is the key for good outcomes.

DISCLOSURE

The authors declare that there are no relevant financial or nonfinancial competing interests to report.

REFERENCES

1. Tamai S, Komatsu S, Sakamoto H, et al. Free muscle transplants in dogs, with microsurgical neurovascular anastomoses. Plast Reconstr Surg 1970;46(3):219–25.
2. Chuang DC. Functioning free-muscle transplantation for the upper extremity. Hand Clin 1997;13(2):279–89.
3. Fischer JP, Elliott RM, Kozin SH, et al. Free function muscle transfers for upper extremity reconstruction: a review of indications, techniques, and outcomes. J Hand Surg 2013;38(12):2485–90.
4. Doi K. Management of total paralysis of the brachial plexus by the double free-muscle transfer technique. J Hand Surg Eur 2008;33(3):240–51.
5. Chuang DC, Strauch RJ, Wei FC. Technical considerations in two-stage functioning free muscle transplantation reconstruction of both flexor and extensor functions of the forearm. Microsurgery 1994;15(5):338–43.
6. Garcia RM, Ruch DS. Free flap functional muscle transfers. Hand Clin 2016;32(3):397–405.
7. Harii K, Ohmori K, Torii S. Free gracilis muscle transplantation, with microneurovascular anastomoses for the treatment of facial paralysis. A preliminary report. Plast Reconstr Surg 1976;57(2):133–43.
8. Free muscle transplantation by microsurgical neurovascular anastomoses. Report of a case. Chin Med J (Engl). 1976;2(1):47–50.
9. Chung KC, Pillsbury MS, Walters MR, et al. Reliability and validity testing of the Michigan hand outcomes Questionnaire. J Hand Surg 1998;23(4):575–87.
10. Zuker RM, Manktelow RT. Functioning free muscle transfers. Hand Clin 2007;23(1):57–72.
11. Seal A, Stevanovic M. Free functional muscle transfer for the upper extremity. Clin Plast Surg 2011;38(4):561–75.

12. Terzis JK, Kostopoulos VK. Free muscle transfer in posttraumatic plexopathies: part III. The hand. Plast Reconstr Surg 2009;124(4):1225–36.

13. Sabapathy SR, Venkatramani H, Bhardwaj P, et al. Technical considerations and outcome of free functioning gracilis muscle transfer for finger flexion in patients with Volkmann's Ischemic Contracture. Injury 2021;52(12):3640–5.

14. Kay S, Pinder R, Wiper J, et al. Microvascular free functioning gracilis transfer with nerve transfer to establish elbow flexion. J Plast Reconstr Aesthetic Surg JPRAS 2010;63(7):1142–9.

15. Griepp DW, Shah NV, Scollan JP, et al. Outcomes of gracilis free-flap muscle transfers and non-free-flap procedures for restoration of elbow flexion: a systematic review. J Plast Reconstr Aesthetic Surg JPRAS 2022;75(8):2625–36.

16. Sechachalam S, O'Byrne A, MacQuillan A. Free functional muscle transfer tendon insertion secondary advancement procedure to improve elbow flexion. Tech Hand Up Extrem Surg 2017;21(1):8–12.

17. Kim JH, Kim I, Seol YJ, et al. Neural cell integration into 3D bioprinted skeletal muscle constructs accelerates restoration of muscle function. Nat Commun 2020;11(1):1025.

18. Doi K, Hattori Y, Soo-Heong T, et al. Endoscopic harvesting of the gracilis muscle for reinnervated free-muscle transfer. Plast Reconstr Surg 1997;100(7):1817–23.

19. Doi K, Arakawa Y, Hattori Y, et al. Restoration of elbow flexion with functioning free muscle transfer in arthrogryposis: a report of two cases. J Bone Joint Surg Am 2011;93(18):e105.

20. Sochol KM, Edwards G, Stevanovic M. Restoration of elbow flexion with a free functional gracilis muscle transfer in an arthrogrypotic patient using a motor nerve to pectoralis major. Hand N Y N 2020;15(5):739–43.

21. Aman M, Boecker AH, Thielen M, et al. Single incision thenar muscle reconstruction using the free functional pronator quadratus flap. BMC Surg 2021;21(1):310.

22. Tadisina KK, Kareh AM, Hasan S, et al. Functional thenar reconstruction: a case report and systematic review of the literature. Ann Plast Surg 2022;89(6):709–15.

Bone Grafts and Flaps in the Management of Complex Upper-Extremity Defects: Indications and Outcomes

Francisco del Piñal, MD, Dr Med

KEYWORDS

- Bone flap • Vascularized bone graft • Vascularized bone phalanx • Finger hand osteomyelitis
- Bone defect in the hand

KEY POINTS

- Most bone defects can be solved by means of nonvascularized bone grafts.
- There is not an upper limit as to when a nonvascularized bone graft will fail.
- Vascularized bone graft is preferred in the context of (1) large bony defect, (2) combined soft tissue defect, (3) infection, (4) poorly vascularized or scarred wound bed, (5) clinical scenario requiring bone and cartilage reconstruction.

INTRODUCTION

Bone defects are a major impediment in upper-limb recovery. Until the underlying bony framework is restored and stable, there is no possibility of appropriate rehabilitation. For this reason, especially in the hand, it is paramount to handle bone defects in an expeditious manner. Obviously, for its simplicity, the ideal is cancellous bone graft. However, the author has a very low threshold for indicating a vascularized bone graft if there are additional complicating factors that may delay healing time and impair function.

From the outset, it should be stated that there *is not* an upper limit as to when a nonvascularized bone graft will fail, and some stunning defects have been solved by this means.[1] However, the surgeon should, at the time of choosing one method or another, take into account the following: (1) the probability of healing, (2) the time it will take (long defects will need months to years to heal), and (3) the morbidity at the donor site (large amounts of iliac crest are not without a price to pay). On the other hand, vascularized bone grafts allow single-stage transport of vast amounts of bone, with minimal healing time. Expedited time to bony union facilitates early rehabilitation, which is critical in the upper limb. The criticism of being a much more complex operation has little sense considering the current expertise in microsurgery in most centers. Hence, in the author's opinion, in an uncomplicated bone defect, the surgeon should lean toward using a bone flap to solve a moderate defect (1.5 cm in the hand and 2.5 cm in the forearm), to speed healing and permit early rehabilitation. Furthermore, if the bed is poor, even minute bony defects are prone to fail if nonvascularized bone grafts are used. Vascularized bone grafts alter the local conditions and can achieve bone healing in the most unfavorable circumstances. Currently, there is general agreement that vascularized bone graft is the best choice when there is a combined soft tissue defect, infection, a poor scarred bed, and when a piece of cartilage needs to be included in the reconstruction.

In this work, the author discusses indications and his favorite bone flaps in the upper limb, after nearly 40 years in the field (**Box 1**). The author stresses that there are hundreds of variations and donor sources, and that some surgeons may think their way/flap is the best; the author does not disagree with that statement.

Hand, Wrist and Microvascular Surgery, Private Practice, Serrano 58-1B, Madrid E-28001, Spain
E-mail address: drpinal@drpinal.com

Clin Plastic Surg 51 (2024) 515–526
https://doi.org/10.1016/j.cps.2024.03.001
0094-1298/24/© 2024 Elsevier Inc. All rights reserved.

> **Box 1**
> **The author's preferred donor bone flaps**
>
> Small defects[a]:
> - Toe phalanx
> - Metatarsal
> - Medial femoral condyle
>
> Long defects:
> - Fibula
> - Scapula
> - Iliac crest
>
> Special needs:
> - Proximal fibula (growing potential)
> - Base of the 3rd metatarsal for radius
> - Trochlea for carpus
>
> [a] Consider also cancellous bone grafts.

NONVASCULARIZED BONE GRAFT

As previously stated, not all bone defects need a flap. Small bone defects, particularly if there is continuity of cortex on one side of the shaft of a phalanx, can be safely grafted with cancellous bone. These defects heal relatively quickly and cause minimal delay in rehabilitation. This is in contrast to structural defects. Gaps larger than 1.5 cm in the metacarpals, or shorter defects in the phalanges, that are less tolerant to immobilization, are better served with one of the bone flaps discussed later.

The volar distal radius is the author's preferred source for cancellous autologous bone graft in the upper limb. Secondarily, the olecranon is a reasonable alternative. Occasionally another place can be the donor site, depending on exposure (**Fig. 1**). There are some limits in the amount of cancellous bone that one can harvest from those donor sites; as stated, the author prefers a vascularized option if the defect is long. The surgeon should take care to pack the cancellous bone tightly. If the defect is small, the author gravitates toward Kirschner wire (K-wire)[2] or intramedullary cannulated screw fixation, rather than plate fixation, in order to minimize soft tissue dissection and provide stability for healing.

VASCULARIZED BONE GRAFT FOR SMALL DEFECTS

The main problem is lack of available donor sites that can reliably carry small segments of structural vascularized bone and a compatible soft tissue paddle. Classic donor sites, such as the fibula or the scapula, are impractical in the hand or fingers. Newer small bone graft donor sites, such as the medial femoral condyle and the modified iliac crest, are unable to carry a flap that matches a soft tissue defect of a finger. For these reasons, the author has implemented the transfer of vascularized toe phalanges.[3,4]

Vascularized Toe Phalanx

Preoperative plain radiographs of bilateral hands and feet (posteroanterior in the standing position) are essential. There is considerable variation in the length of the middle phalanx among patients and, at times, between the 2 feet (**Fig. 2**).

As a rule, the middle phalanx is the preferred donor site because it affords a longer pedicle. Before its takeoff from the intermetatarsal arteries, the arterial pedicle can be dissected 3 to 4 cm proximally. This is sufficient to carry the anastomosis to a digital artery in the hand, away from the immediate area of injury. Conversely, the proximal phalanx, especially if the base is to be harvested, yields a much shorter pedicle (1–1.5 cm of proper digital artery), unless the dissection proceeds proximally on one of the metatarsal arteries. Inclusion of the parent metatarsal artery may not be beneficial, owing to the possibility of significant size mismatch with the recipient digital artery. Furthermore, the surgeon would need to perform additional dissection, increasing the risk of vascular spasm and operative time. Adept microsurgical technique is a prerequisite, as the caliber of the toe digital arteries is typically 0.5 to 1 mm.

The blood supply to the toe phalanges is rarely dependent on a single nutrient artery, but on tiny periosteal and capsular branches arising from the digital arteries. Two constant arcades encircle the neck of the proximal phalanx and the base of the middle phalanx. At the base of the proximal phalanx, osseous branches derive from the plantar and dorsal digital.[5,6]

The procedure is similar to a standard toe harvest, with some particularities highlighted in late discussion.[7] The skin flap is designed over the bone to be harvested. Through a dorsal zigzag incision, a subcutaneous vein is first dissected and isolated. The skin flap is incised on the side of the pedicle and elevated plantarward. Great care is essential to keep intact the connections between the digital artery, the donor bone, and the vein dorsally. Including a soft tissue cuff in the vicinity of the bone helps protect the vascularity. The corresponding digital nerve is dissected away from the digital artery, reflected plantarly and left on the toe. The digital artery is the

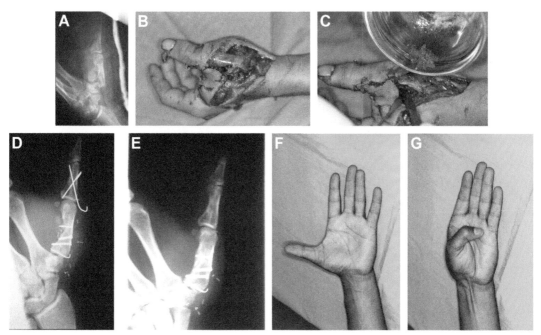

Fig. 1. (*A*) This 22-year-old patient sustained an open fracture with bone loss in the first metacarpal. (*B*) After debridement and bony stabilization, coverage was planned with a lateral arm free flap. (*C*) A substantial amount of cancellous bone was harvested from the epicondyle, to solve a defect of two-thirds of the circumference of the metacarpal (*D*). (*E–G*) Radiograph showing the bony healing and result at 10 years. (*Courtesy of* Dr Piñal, MD, Dr. Med. 2023.)

dissected proximally, and side branches are tied off with 5-0 silk, clips, or 9-0 nylon, depending on their size. Traction on these tiny branches is to be avoided, as avulsion from the main digital artery may cause persistent spasm or even failure of the part to be revascularized.[8] The digital artery is ligated distal to the bone to be harvested.

Once the dissection on the pedicle's side is terminated, the contralateral side is rapidly dissected out by incising the skin island and performing a subperiosteal dissection of the phalanx. The neurovascular pedicle, that would maintain the donor toe viability, does not actually need to be seen. Only nutrient branches to the bone from this pedicle need to be carefully ligated, again avoiding avulsion, as this may endanger the toe's blood supply. The flexor sheath is opened, and the flexor tendons are reflected plantarward. Care should be taken not to avulse the vincular tissue, as this may damage the tiny rete of vessels located along the plantar aspect of the phalanx. The segment of bone to be harvested is then cut, and the tourniquet is released. The author tries to cut the exact amount of bone needed before disconnecting the phalanx from the toe, as afterward it is very difficult to manipulate the small block of bone. The flap is then ready to be transferred and revascularized in the usual way (**Fig. 3**).

The donor site is closed primarily in all cases. The donor site bone defect is partially closed by axial collapse and by suturing the extensor to the flexor tendons. This is performed in a similar manner to the technique used in pediatric nonvascularized proximal phalanx harvest. The toe is preserved in all cases and remains vascularized by the contralateral pedicle (**Fig. 4**).

Once the blood supply has been demonstrated in the foot, the flap is transferred to the hand. In most cases the bone is fixed with crossed 1.0-mm K-wires, to reduce the interference with the blood supply and also to minimize hardware in infected beds. Revascularization is end to end to a digital artery in all cases. In most cases, the author tries to do flow-through configurations. Venous drainage is accomplished by anastomosing a dorsal vein end to end to a subcutaneous vein in the digital web. In most cases, continuous 10-0 nylon (on a 100-μ needle) was used for the arteries and continuous 9-0 nylon (on a 150-μ needle) was used for the veins. Transitory spasm is quite common when dealing with very small vessels (toe digital arteries are in the range of 0.6–1.2 mm). If present, vasospasm can be treated with topical agents, such as verapamil or papaverine. In addition, just before clamps release, the author administers a bolus of 1500 U of heparin

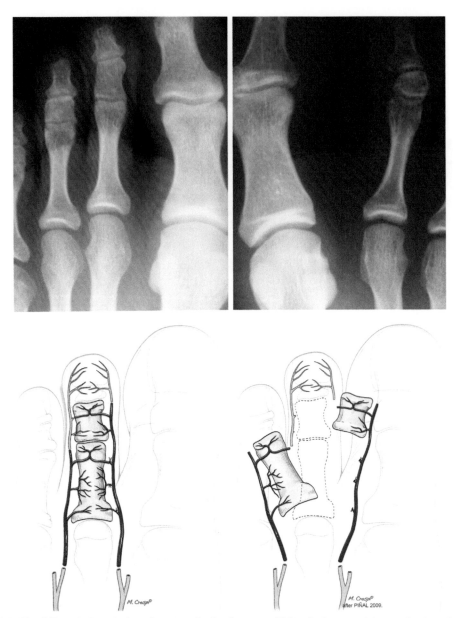

Fig. 2. Considerable variations in length may exist in the toe middle phalanx, and it may be too short to be useable. (*bottom*) However, the middle phalanx is the author's preferred choice. It provides the longest pedicle, and the donor site can be closed by shortening arthroplasty. (*Courtesy of* Dr Piñal MD, Dr. Med. 2011.)

intravenously. Thereafter, a continuous perfusion of heparin (500 U of heparin per hour) is administered for the first 2 days, followed by 250 U per hour for an additional 2 days. Patients are discharged on day 3 to 4 on low-molecular-weight heparin, for an average of 2 weeks or less pending ambulatory status. Patients are allowed to walk in a postoperative stiff-sole shoe after 2 or 3 days. Clinical bone union occurred in all cases earlier than 4 weeks. In uncomplicated cases, antibiotics are stopped on postoperative day 5. In the setting

of infection, narrow- or broad-spectrum antibiotics are administered for 6 weeks (in most cases a quinolone plus rifampicin).

Vascularized Metatarsal

The metatarsal has a nutrient foramen at the distal third[5,9] and also a rich periosteal network dependent on the plantar and dorsal metatarsal arteries.[9] This vascular disposition allows safe harvest of a portion of the lateral aspect of the first metatarsal,

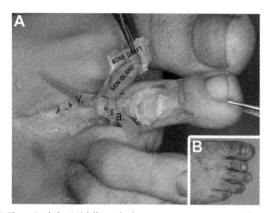

Fig. 3. (A) Middle phalanx osteocutaneous flap elevated and pedicled on its vascular axis before tourniquet release (a, lateral plantar digital artery of the second toe; v, subcutaneous vein). Notice that the digital nerve is not included with the flap but preserved on the toe. (B) (inset) Result at 1 year. (The hallux nail deformity depends on a recent unrelated trauma.). (*Courtesy of* Dr Piñal MD, Dr. Med. 2008.)

a portion of the medial aspect of the second metatarsal, or the whole of the second metatarsal.[10] The author has experience on both hemi-first metatarsal and -second metatarsal, although the

former has been surpassed, by far, by the medial femoral condyle (see later discussion).

Flap elevation is similar to the technique for harvest of a dorsalis pedis, except that a piece of metatarsal is included in this case.[11] If the second metatarsal is to be fully harvested, the dorsalis pedicle is identified proximal to the web and traced distally to the takeoff of the deep plantar artery, at the most proximal aspect of the web. The origin of the first dorsal metatarsal (FDMA) is identified here and dissected out. Adjacent to the bone to be harvested, all soft tissue lateral to the artery is left intact to protect the tiny periosteal vessels going to the metatarsal. Once the medial part of the dissection is finished, the lateral aspect of the metatarsal is defined, preserving only the periosteum of the bone, if the whole circumference is to be included. In the case of a hemi-metatarsal, the dissection is carried over the dorsal aspect of the metatarsal while keeping intact the medial attachments to the bone. The flap is now elevated, and the tourniquet is released to ascertain that the bone has adequate vascularity.

The author has always included a small skin island for covering, filling of dead space, and monitoring purposes. If a skin island is needed, it

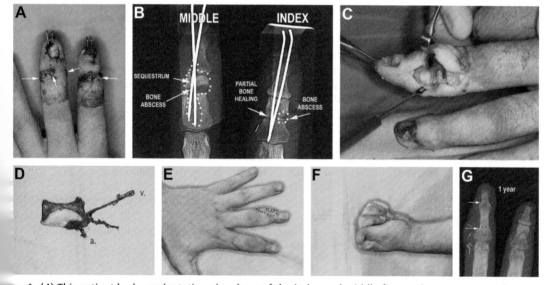

Fig. 4. (A) This patient had a replantation elsewhere of the index and middle finger. The patient came for a second opinion, as he was scheduled for a secondary amputation. Multiple draining sinuses were present in the middle finger and in the radial aspect of the index (arrows). (B) On the radiographs, the index presented a radial abscess and a partially healed fracture ulnarly. A massive abscess was present in the middle finger with the distal proximal phalanx acting as a sequestrum. (C) After debridement, the middle finger had a through-and-through soft tissue defect and a bone defect that involved most of the middle phalanx and the distal interphalangeal joint. (D) A vascularized second toe proximal phalanx spanned the bony ends. Notice that minimal fixation was used to stabilize this vascularized bone graft. The index hardware was left in place, as it was away from the infection. However, the bone was debrided; cancellous bone was applied, and a local flap (a hatchet flap) was used for coverage. No other surgery had been performed. (E and F) Functional range of motion of the proximal interphalangeal joint was achieved. (G) Plain radiographs showed complete bone healing of the toe phalanx (arrows). Infection has not recurred after 6 years. (*Courtesy of* Dr Piñal MD, Dr. Med. 2015.)

should be borne in mind that, although acceptable for a metacarpal, it will be slightly bulky for a finger. In addition, unless a medium-size flap is to be included (that can be designed on the axis of the FDMA), a specific cutaneous perforator should be isolated and traced. Not doing so risks compromising the skin island. Technically, this is quite demanding. To accommodate variations, the author first incises one side of the skin island and adjusts the island's location, according to where a sizable skin perforator is located.

The flap is unusable if the FDMA artery is absent (Gilbert type III).[12] Moreover, although the bony portion will be vascularized when the FDMA is located deep between the interosseous muscles (Gilbert type II), the cutaneous paddle will not, and use of the flap will be impracticable. Based on the author's experience with toe harvesting, he has noticed that Doppler is very helpful to define when the FDMA is absent. It is, however, unable to differentiate a medium-size superficially located FDMA from a normal-size, but deep, FDMA. Therefore, if there is a preoperative doubt about its presence, the author thinks it is wiser to try the other foot or a different donor site.

Traditionally, the dorsalis pedis is considered a second-line flap owing to its significant donor site if a large skin flap is required. This is usually not the case for this specific application, and minimal morbidity exists when only a portion of a metatarsal is harvested. The second toe may need to be removed if a large amount of bone is needed. Alternatively, the digit can be syndactylized to the third toe by creating a bony bar. In summary, the indications for this flap are limited, but it is ideal for a large defect in any metacarpal (**Fig. 5**). Massive defects involving several metacarpals are better solved with an iliac crest bone graft[13] or variations of a double-barrel fibula (see later discussion).[14]

Corticoperiosteal Flap

Periosteal flaps in theory are ideal as they adapt well to hand defects without providing bulkiness. Unfortunately, the initial results of transferring vascularized periosteum were inconsistent.[15] Sakai and colleagues[16] realized that harvesting the periosteum alone would damage the "cambium layer" (the deepest layer of the periosteum where most osteoblasts are located), endangering the ability of the transferred periosteum to form bone. However, when a thin layer of external cortex of the femur is included, the flap maintains its bone-forming ability.

The corticoperiosteal flap from the medial condyle has proved successful in difficult cases.[17,18] It

should be stressed that bony bridges could be seen on radiographs as early as 6 to 8 weeks after flap transfer in patients that had had up to 7 previous operations. Although Sakai and coworkers[16] advised thinning the bone component of the flap, for adaptation to complex defects, this has the disadvantage of reducing the vascularized bone transferred and also risks damaging the periosteum. The author prefers to harvest a thicker layer of cancellous bone (about 3 mm thick). The cortical bone is cut with an oscillating saw, maintaining the periosteum so that it will act as a hinge (**Fig. 6**). In this way, a larger volume of vascularized bone is included, and there is less risk of damaging the periosteum. This bone growth can be explained by the high osteogenic, osteoinductive, and osteoblastic capacity of the periosteal flap.[19] By wrapping the corticoperiosteal flap around the nonunion on the side opposite to the plate, the nonunion can be almost surrounded by well-vascularized, bone-forming tissue.[17,18]

Once the intricacies of the anatomy are understood, the flap is extremely easy to raise. The author routinely performs flap harvest in 20 minutes or less. Upper-extremity indications for this have surged since inception, although the excitement must be accompanied by some restraint. Too large a flap can cause a femoral condyle fracture of disastrous consequences.[20] The author limits the flap size to 4 × 4 cm and harvests it in the condyle itself, ending distal to the flare of the metaphysis. The author harvests some amount of cancellous bone graft as well.

The main indication for this flap is to achieve union in complex malunions or nonunions of the scaphoid, in metacarpals nonunions or infected beds (**Fig. 7**), and in difficult or failed intercarpal arthrodesis.[21,22] Segmental defects in the forearm and arm, or difficult nonunions, can be solved in one stage with this flap.[16–18,21] The author does not use this flap in any defect larger than 3 cm (note that a part of the flap needs to overlap the recipient one) for fear of having a major complication.

VASCULARIZED BONE GRAFTS FOR LARGER DEFECTS

Although alternative vascularized bone flaps can be used, such as iliac crest or scapular bone undoubtably, the fibula is the king of the larger defects group (more than 5 cm) and is the only option if the defect is greater than 10 cm.[13,23] The flap was described by Taylor and colleagues[24] and has evolved dramatically since its inception, with regards to dissection technique and the inclusion of a skin flap with the bone.[25]

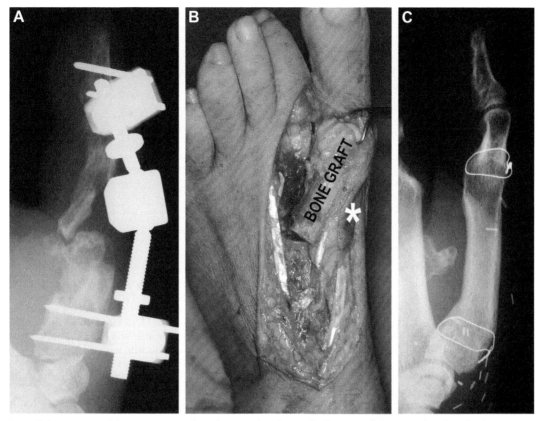

Fig. 5. (*A*) A 52-year-old patient was referred 3 months after suffering a crush injury to his thumb. The proximal pins were discharging pus too. In a single stage, the infected scarred tissues (including the infected proximal pin tracks) were excised. (*B*) A 5-cm segment of metatarsal was used to span the defect. A skin monitor is marked with an asterisk. (*C*) The patient has been free of infection for 10 years. (*Courtesy of* Dr Piñal MD, Dr. Med. 2008.)

The flap is usually based on the peroneal vessels, and the dissection technique is well known. The reader is referred to other sources for further details.[26] Nonetheless, apart from simple defects, the refinements on the insetting allows daring configurations and solves "impossible" defects (**Figs. 8 and 9**).[14,26,27]

SPECIALIZED BONE DEFECTS
Epiphyseal Transfer: Proximal Fibula

Taylor and colleagues[28] described for the first time the possibility of transplanting a piece of fibula with growth potential. Innocenti and colleagues[29] based the elevation of the flap on the anterior recurrent artery, refined the harvesting technique,

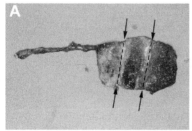 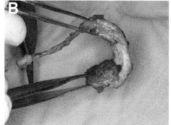 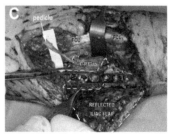

Fig. 6. Tailoring the corticoperiosteal flap. (*A*) Two parallel cuts in the surface (bony side) of the flap (*arrows*) had been made with an oscillating saw, taking care not to penetrate the periosteum. (*B*) After the osteotomy, the cortical segments can easily be rotated through 90° on the intact periosteum, which acts as a hinge to be wrapped around the defect in the ulna opposite to the plate (*C*). C-P, corticoperiosteal flap. (*Courtesy of* Dr Piñal MD, Dr. Med. 2015.)

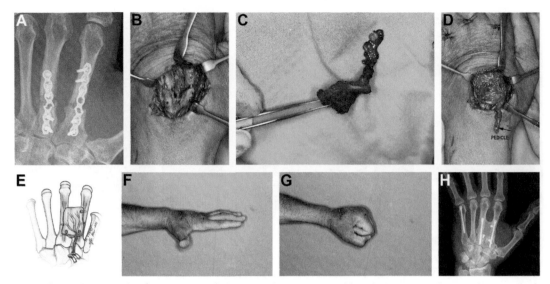

Fig. 7. This patient sustained an open crush injury and was managed by plating. According to the report, the intrinsic muscles were devitalized and had to be debrided. All these unfavorable factors led to an atrophic nonunion and hardware failure (*A*). To overcome an exhausted bed (with no healing potential) (*B*) apart from a new fixation, vascularized tissue with osteogenic potential was planned. (See the cannulated screws in the medullary canal.) (*C*) A wedge-shaped flap from the medial femoral condyle was harvested and fixed in position with lag screws (*D* and *E*). In the same surgery, tenolysis and capsulotomies (second to fourth) were added to treat the stiff hand. (*F* and *G*) Immediate range of motion was started, and a full functional result was achieved at 3 weeks. (*H*) Final radiograph at 10 years. (*Courtesy of* Dr Piñal MD, Dr. Med. 2015.)

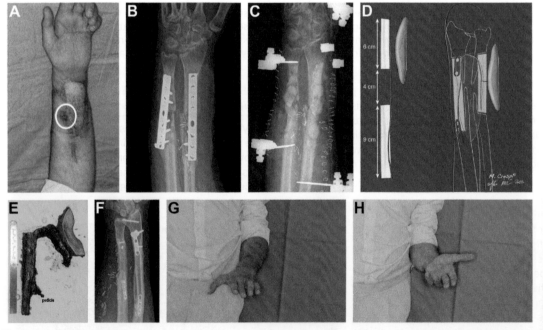

Fig. 8. (*A*) This 24-year-old patient sustained an open fracture to radius and ulna 5 months before being under the care of the author. At that time, a draining sinus (*circle*) and loosening of the hardware are evident. (*B*) The radius and ulna were radically debrided, and the antibiotic-impregnated cement beads, acting as a spacer, were left for a week (*C*). (*D*) The planned surgery and the corresponding fibula flap with the skin island in the distal bony segment (*E*). (*F*) Radiograph 3 years after the reconstruction. (*G* and *H*) The patient achieved nearly full pronosupination stressing the importance of this double-barreled reconstruction instead of a single-bone forearm. (*Courtesy of* Dr Piñal MD, Dr. Med. 2020.)

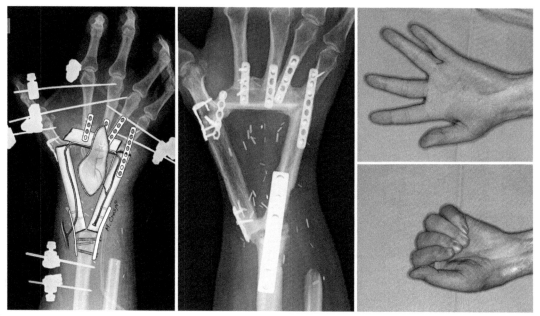

Fig. 9. A 10-cm defect after resection of a tumor in the carpus was solved by a delta-shaped fibula in one stage. (*right*) The patient is free of disease 10 years after the reconstruction. (*Courtesy of* Dr Piñal MD, Dr. Med. 2021.)

and presented impressive series. The harvesting technique is complex, and there may be the need for cutting the motor branch to the anterior tibial muscle. This usually recovers in 3 to 5 months, although this recovery period is certainly a major source of stress for the family and surgeon. This should be emphasized to the family, as the flap is unsurpassed by other alternatives and is a single-stage solution to complex problems (**Fig. 10**).

Osteochondral Flaps

In some cases where cartilage has been irreversibly damaged in the radius, the base of the third metatarsal has been transferred successfully to restore a gliding cartilaginous surface.[30] The indications are limited, and the author is leaning more and more toward using a combination of arthroscopic-guided osteotomy and arthroscopic resection arthroplasty.[31,32] However, there is no operation that can compete with this technique, when there is damage to the lunate facet and the sigmoid notch. In these instances, the base of the third metatarsal is unsurpassed by morbid alternatives, including partial carpal fusion (for the radius facet) and a Darrach or a distal radioulnar joint prosthesis (**Fig. 11**).[33]

Flap harvesting

There is a competitive situation in the blood supply the base of the third metatarsal.[30,33] The dominant blood supply is either the arcuate artery or the distal lateral tarsal artery, both branches of the dorsalis pedis-FDMA artery. The surgeon must expose the base of the metatarsal and choose the larger vessel. Although apparently frightening not knowing the dominant vessel, most perforators flaps are the same way (freestyle), so this should not cause much hesitation when choosing this flap. In all the author's cases, the dominant vessel was tracked to the larger dorsalis pedis, without significant microsurgical difficulties. The venous drainage is via the venae comitantes in all cases. Further details can be found in the original papers.

Other Osteochondral Donor Sites

Small defects in the critical carpal bones have been solved by using variations of the vascularized osteochondral graft concept described earlier. The femoral trochlea is the most popular flap for those scenarios.[34,35] Nevertheless, complex problems may call for sophisticated flap designs with the same principles.[36,37]

The main indication for the popular medial (or lateral) trochlea flap is for proximal pole scaphoid nonunions. From the author's perspective as a hand surgeon, the ligaments joining the scaphoid to the lunate are left unrepaired in most cases, and that may create a situation similar to a scapholunate dissociation in the mid term. Also, the author has had patients complaining of knee

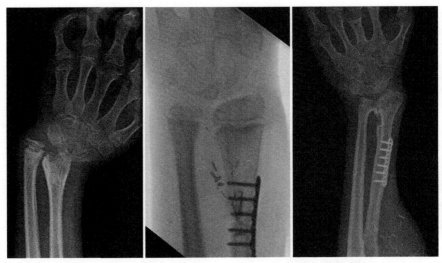

Fig. 10. This 12-year-old boy suffered a congenital Volkmann. Apart from the muscle damage and the general severe growth disturbance of the limb, the radius distal epiphysis was more severely affected with a radial collapse of the hand. A proximal fibula epiphysis was transferred (*center*). The result at the end of the growth is shown on the right.

pain, although this is rare. Despite its elegance, in the author's armamentarium, the indications for this flap are limited to cases where other more classic alternatives (arthroscopic bone grafting or fusions) have no role. Perhaps Preiser and noncollapsed Kienböck disease are the ideal instances for this flap. Nevertheless, Bürger and colleagues[34] and others have found much wider indications and reported satisfactory results. The reader is referred to those studies.[34,35,38]

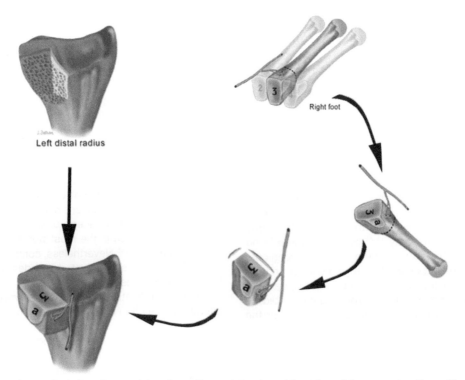

Left distal radius

Right foot

Fig. 11. Defect in the left radius involving the radius and the sigmoid notch and the reconstruction with a vascularized osteochondral graft of the base of the third metatarsal.

DISCUSSION

Bone flaps offer a solution to complex situations and large bone defects. In the setting of infection, especially with long-standing osteomyelitis, proper debridement and wound bed preparation are of equal importance. The bone is approached through the wound itself in the acute situation and through the sinus and/or previous scars in cases of chronic osteomyelitis. The sinus is excised, and any marginally viable tissue is removed en bloc. Granulating, scarred, or devitalized soft tissue is excised. Deep cultures are taken from the bone and deep granulation tissue. Bone is excised until clearly viable healthy tissue is found, which is the single most important step of this procedure. Ideally, before this stage, no antibiotics are given. However, most cases have previously failed courses of antibiotics prescribed by referring physicians. The tourniquet is deflated at this stage to ensure bleeding from the bone.

Flap fixation is challenging. The goal is to provide sufficient fixation while avoiding any disruption to the blood supply. Fixation depends on surgeon preference, and the author is aware that well-known surgeons prefer rigid fixation with large AO plates to provide immediate stability.[26] The author prefers smaller plates and alternative means of fixation, including external fixation in some cases, to disturb the bony blood supply as minimally as possible.

In summary, bone flaps are extremely useful when spanning bone defects in complicated beds, in the upper limb. They are first line, in the author's experience, in defects longer than 1 cm in the phalanges and 3 cm in the forearm bones.

CLINICS CARE POINTS

- Vascularized bone flaps are extremely useful tools when spanning bone defects in the upper limb in complicated beds.

- The surgeon should lean toward using a bone flap to solve a moderate defect to speed healing and permit early rehabilitation.

- Bone flaps are first choice in the author's experience in defects longer than 1 cm in the phalanges and 3 cm in the forearm bones.

DISCLOSURE

The author has nothing to disclose.

REFERENCES

1. Ring D, Jupiter JB. Wave plate osteosynthesis in the upper extremity. Tech Hand Up Extrem Surg 1997; 1(3):168–74.

2. Piñal Matorras F del, Cruz Cámara A, Serrano Criado A, et al. "Fijación interna mínima y espongio-plastia inmediata" en fracturas abiertas conminutas del pulgar. Cir Plast Iberlatinamer 1999;25:99–105 [Spanish].

3. del Piñal F, Moraleda E, Rúas JS, et al. Minimally invasive fixation of fractures of the phalanges and metacarpals with intramedullary cannulated headless compression screws. J Hand Surg Am 2015; 40(4):692–700.

4. del Piñal F, García-Bernal FJ, Delgado J, et al. Vascularized bone blocks from the toe phalanx to solve complex intercalated defects in the fingers. J Hand Surg Am 2006;31(7):1075–82.

5. Yoshizu T, Watanabe M, Tajima T. Étude expérimentale et applications cliniques des transferts libres d'articulation d'orteil avec anastomoses vasculaires. In: Tubiana R, editor. Traité de chirurgie de la main, 2. Paris: Masson; 1984. p. 539–51.

6. Chen YG, Cook PA, McClinton MA, et al. Microarterial anatomy of the lesser toe proximal interphalangeal joints. J Hand Surg Am 1998;23(2): 256–60.

7. Piñal F del. The indications for toe transfer after "minor" finger injuries. J Hand Surg [Br] 2004;29:120–9.

8. Del Piñal F, García-Bernal FJ, Ayala H, et al. Ischemic toe encountered during harvesting: report of 6 cases. J Hand Surg Am 2008;33(10):1820–5.

9. Shereff MJ, Yang QM, Kummer FJ. Extraosseous and intraosseous arterial supply to the first metatarsal and metatarsophalangeal joint. Foot Ankle 1987;8:81–93.

10. MacLeod AM, Robinson DW. Reconstruction of defects involving the mandible and floor of mouth by free osteo-cutaneous flaps derived from the foot. Br J Plast Surg 1982;35:239–46.

11. Man D, Acland RD. The microarterial anatomy of the dorsalis pedis flap and its clinical applications. Plast Reconstr Surg 1980;65:419–23.

12. Gilbert A. Composite tissue transfer from the foot: anatomic basis and surgical technique. In: Daniller AJ, Strauch B, editors. Symposium on microsurgery. St Louis: Mosby; 1976. p. 230–42.

13. Taylor GI, Townsend P, Corlett R. Superiority of the deep circumflex iliac vessels as the supply for free groin flaps. Clinical work. Plast Reconstr Surg 1979;64(6):745–59.

14. Jones NF, Swartz WM, Mears DC, et al. The "double barrel" free vascularized fibular bone graft. Plast Reconstr Surg 1988;81:378–85.

15. Romaña MC, Masquelet AC. Vascularized periosteum associated with cancellous bone graft: an

experimental study. Plast Reconstr Surg 1990;85(4):587–92.

16. Sakai K, Doi K, Kawai S. Free vascularized thin corticoperiosteal graft. Plast Reconstr Surg 1991;87:290–8.

17. Del Piñal F. An Update on the management of severe crush injury to the forearm and hand. Clin Plast Surg 2020;47(4):461–89.

18. Del Piñal F, García-Bernal FJ, Regalado J, et al. Vascularised corticoperiosteal grafts from the medial femoral condyle for difficult non-unions of the upper limb. J Hand Surg Eur 2007;32(2):135–42.

19. Vögelin E, Jones NF, Huang JI, et al. Healing of a critical-sized defect in the rat femur with use of a vascularized periosteal flap, a biodegradable matrix, and bone morphogenetic protein. J Bone Joint Surg Am 2005;87(6):1323–31.

20. Son JH, Giladi AM, Higgins JP. Iatrogenic femur fracture following medial femoral condyle flap harvest eventually requiring total knee arthroplasty in one patient. J Hand Surg Eur 2019;44(3):320–1.

21. Doi K, Oda T, Soo-Heong T, et al. Free vascularized bone graft for nonunion of the scaphoid. J Hand Surg Am 2000;25(3):507–19.

22. Del Piñal F, Studer A, Thams C, et al. Sigmoid notch reconstruction and limited carpal arthrodesis for a severely comminuted distal radius malunion: case report. J Hand Surg Am 2012;37(3):481–5.

23. Sekiguchi J, Kobayashi S, Ohmori K. Use of the osteocutaneous free scapular flap on the lower extremities. Plast Reconstr Surg 1993;91(1):103–12.

24. Taylor GI, Miller GD, Ham FJ. The free vascularized bone graft. A clinical extension of microvascular techniques. Plast Reconstr Surg 1975;55(5):533–44.

25. Wei FC, Chen HC, Chuang CC, et al. Fibular osteoseptocutaneous flap: anatomic study and clinical application. Plast Reconstr Surg 1986;78(2):191–200.

26. del Piñal F, Innocenti M. Evolving concepts in the management of the bone gap in the upper limb. Long and small defects. J Plast Reconstr Aesthet Surg 2007;60(7):776–92.

27. Graham D, Sivakumar B, Piñal FD. Triangular vascularized free fibula flap for massive carpal reconstruction. J Hand Surg Am 2022;47(2):196.e1–6.

28. Taylor GI, Wilson KR, Rees MD, et al. The anterior tibial vessels and their role in epiphyseal and diaphyseal transfer of the fibula: experimental study and clinical applications. Br J Plast Surg 1988 Sep;41(5):451–69.

29. Innocenti M, Delcroix L, Manfrini M, et al. Vascularized proximal fibular epiphyseal transfer for distal radial reconstruction. J Bone Joint Surg Am 2005;87(Suppl 1):237–46.

30. Del Piñal F, García-Bernal FJ, Delgado J, et al. Reconstruction of the distal radius facet by a free vascularized osteochondral autograft: anatomic study and report of a patient. J Hand Surg Am 2005;30(6):1200–10.

31. del Piñal F, García-Bernal FJ, Delgado J, et al. Correction of malunited intra-articular distal radius fractures with an inside-out osteotomy technique. J Hand Surg Am 2006;31(6):1029–34.

32. del Piñal F, Klausmeyer M, Thams C, et al. Arthroscopic resection arthroplasty for malunited intra-articular distal radius fractures. J Hand Surg Am 2012;37(12):2447–55.

33. del Piñal F, Klausmeyer M, Moraleda E, et al. Vascularized graft from the metatarsal base for reconstructing major osteochondral distal radius defects. J Hand Surg Am 2013;38(10):1883–95.

34. Bürger HK, Windhofer C, Gaggl AJ, et al. Vascularized medial femoral trochlea osteocartilaginous flap reconstruction of proximal pole scaphoid nonunions. J Hand Surg Am 2013;38(4):690–700.

35. Higgins JP, Bürger HK. Medial femoral trochlea osteochondral flap: applications for scaphoid and lunate reconstruction. Clin Plast Surg 2017;44(2):257–65.

36. del Piñal F, Guerrero-Navarro ML, Studer A, et al. Reconstruction of the ulnar head with a vascularized second metatarsal head: case report. J Hand Surg Am 2012;37(8):1568–73.

37. Del Piñal F, Cromheecke M, Chaves C. Free vascularized second metatarsophalangeal joint transfer for scaphotrapezial joint reconstruction after distal scaphoid excision and carpal collapse: a case report. Microsurgery 2022;42(3):282–6.

38. Windhofer CM, Higgins JP, Gaggl A, et al. Lateral femoral trochlea osteochondral flap reconstruction of proximal Pole scaphoid nonunions. J Hand Surg Am 2022;1. S0363-5023(22)00505-6.

Dupuytren's Contracture
Approach to Treatment and Counseling Patients in 2024

Anthony M. Kordahi, MD[a], Jignesh V. Unadkat, MD[a],*

KEYWORDS

- Dupuytren • Dupuytren's • Contracture • Needle aponeurotomy • Palmar fasciectomy
- Collagenase

KEY POINTS

- Dupuytren disease is a progressive disease that causes debilitating flexion contractures of the metacarpophalangeal and proximal interphalangeal joints.
- There are a range of treatment options from minimally invasive to surgical excision of the pathologic tissue.
- Our understanding of the disease process continues to evolve. Depending on the extent of flexion contracture, needle aponeurotomy and collagenase injection have satisfactory results with moderate long-term efficacy.
- Surgical palmar fasciectomy continues to be the gold standard for extensive contracture and long-standing results.

NATURE OF THE PROBLEM/DEFINITIONS

Dupuytren disease (DD) is a benign fibroproliferative disorder of the palmar and digital fascia. It is characterized by contracted longitudinal cords and discrete nodules. The shortening of these contracted tissues along lines of mechanical tension causes contractures of the metacarpophalangeal (MCP) and proximal interphalangeal (PIP) joints and subsequent functional impairment. Pathologic cords displace neurovascular (NV) structures in the palm and digits, further complicating intervention. This result of DD is called Dupuytren contracture (DC).[1]

Classically, staging for DC was put forth by Tubiana as follows:

0 No lesion
N Palmar nodule without the presence of contracture

1 Total flexion deformity between 0° and 45°
2 Total flexion deformity between 45° and 90°
3 Total flexion deformity between 90° and 135°
4 Total flexion deformity greater than 135°[2]

PATHOGENESIS/GENETICS

The precise pathogenesis of DD has yet to be fully elucidated. It has long been believed to be a disease of the Vikings, with northern European origination. Mean prevalence in Western countries is 12% at age 55 years, 21% at age 65 years, and 29% at age 75 years.[3] Less than one-fifth of all patients with DD progress to develop DCs.[4] Inheritance studies demonstrate an autosomal dominant pattern with variable penetrance.[5] The evolving body of literature demonstrates that while DD affects Asians, Hispanics, and Africans, its prevalence is greatest among Caucasians.[6]

a Division of Plastic Surgery, University of Chicago, The University of Chicago Medicine & Biological Sciences, 5841 South Maryland Avenue, Room J641, Chicago, IL 60637, USA
* Corresponding author.
E-mail address: Jignesh.unakdat@bsd.uchicago.edu

Clin Plastic Surg 51 (2024) 527–537
https://doi.org/10.1016/j.cps.2024.05.002

The strongest indicator of disease likelihood is a positive family background. Family history is associated with an earlier onset of the disease and earlier initiation of treatment. Research indicates that having a family history involving both parents with the condition usually leads to an earlier onset than if only one parent is affected. Furthermore, the presence of an affected sibling notably increases the risk of developing the disease. Men are 7 to 15 times more likely than women to require surgery for DD. Women develop the condition later in life and experience a more benign course of the disease than men.[7] While these observations strongly point toward a genetic connection, a particular genetic location associated with the disease remains unidentified.[8]

A large volume of evidence has been published on the associations with DD, including tobacco use, alcohol use, diabetes, regional trauma, and heavy manual labor. However, no studies have been able to identify a comorbidity or predisposition with direct causation. DD does not appear to be a monoclonal process. In particular, proteins involved in the Wnt-signaling pathway have been identified as being profibrotic within DD.[9] Studies evaluating the human leucocyte antigen (HLA) status of individuals with DD have demonstrated an increased incidence of HLA-DRB1*01 genotype in Caucasians with DD, and HLA-B7 haplotype in both Peyronie's disease and DD.[10] Lesions of DD show increased amounts of type III collagen and many of the biochemical features of granulation and scar tissue.[11]

Dupuytren diathesis represents an aggressive variant of disease with worse outcomes. The presence of rapidly progressing contractures in a young individual signals a robust "Dupuytren's predisposition," as outlined by Hueston and Mac-Callum. A strong predisposition is identifiable in a patient who meets specific criteria: a significant family history, an early onset of the condition, bilateral affliction (especially affecting the radial side of the hand), widespread involvement with the skin, and abnormal deposits found in areas like the soles of the feet (Ledderhose disease), the penis (Peyronie's disease), or over the back of the PIP joints (Garrod knuckle pads). Of significance is the quick reappearance of symptoms following fasciectomy, which indicates a powerful predisposition.[12]

NORMAL ANATOMY

The superficial palmar fascia is a triangular-shaped collection of longitudinal fibers that divide into a central pretendinous band extending into each of the fingers. The thumb does not contain a central band of fascial tissue. The superficial transverse palmar ligament connects the central bands at the level of the distal palmar crease. From this point, the central pretendinous bands trifurcate. The superficial fibers merge with vertical retinacular fibers at the undersurface of the dermis. The intermediate fibers are known as the spiral band and cause particular disturbance to the NV bundle. Proximally, these fibers lie central and superficial to the bundle, while distally, they exist lateral and deep to the bundle. Deep fibers travel dorsally through the transverse metacarpal ligament and merge with the fibers of the sagittal band.[1,13]

The web spaces between the fingers contain transverse and obliquely oriented fibers named natatory ligaments. These fibers continue laterally to contribute to Greyson's ligaments as well as to attach to the underside of the dermis. The digital fascial network consists of a meshwork of layers of fibers that exist to maintain the rotatory stability of the digital skin in relation to the underlying structures. The network of fibers dorsal to the NV bundle are termed Cleland ligaments, while those volar to the NV are termed Greyson's ligaments. Further, on the ulnar aspect of the small finger, the abductor digiti minimi fascia and tendon contain attachments that run longitudinally along the finger as well as toward the skin.[14]

PATHOLOGIC ANATOMY

The normally supple fascial bands and connective tissue described in the previous section become thickened and firm in DD. This thickening results in bands turning into cords, resulting in the clinical manifestations found in DC. In the process of cord formation, there is a reorientation of collagen fibers parallel to lines of mechanical stress. The central pretendinous bands undergo biological changes similar to those experienced in wound healing. There is an increased amount of type III collagen deposition with pathologic features similar to those of scar tissue.[11] These thickened pretendinous bands are then termed pretendinous cords. They may cause MCP joint flexion as the pretendinous cords cross the MCP flexion crease to coalesce with the pathologic spiral cords and lateral digital sheets. The NV bundles are not displaced by the pretendinous cords; thus, when releasing isolated MCP joint contractures, the digital arteries and nerves should not be at risk.

Continuing past the MCP joint into the finger, the pathologic spiral cord contains fibers of the spiral band, lateral digital sheet, and Greyson's ligaments. In the small finger, particularly, it may arise from the intrinsic tendon, such as the abductor digiti minimi.[15] As the contracture progresses, the fibers of the spiral cord shorten and straighten. This displaces the NV bundle more superficially, and toward the midline of the finger, placing it at risk during surgical dissection (**Fig. 1**). Spiral NV bundles have been reported in up to half of all DD patients. This displacement is most commonly located between the level of the distal palmar crease and the flexion crease of the PIP joint.[16] Three digital cords exist: central, lateral, and spiral, and they all have insertions onto the flexor sheath and middle phalanx. The majority of PIP contractures is due to multiple digital cords, which, in order of frequency, are central digital, retrovascular, and spiral or lateral.[17]

Minimizing stress on specific areas leads to a reduction in the risk of contracture in certain locations. Structures rarely affected due to stress shielding include the Cleland ligament, which is guarded by the adjacent phalanx; the longitudinal fibers beneath the transverse superficial palmar ligament, which is protected by the central band; the transverse superficial palmar ligament, which is shielded by the transverse metacarpal ligament; and the septa of Legueu and Juvara, which are shielded by the adjacent metacarpal. Stress shielding also marks the endpoint of disease progression. As capsuloligamentous joint contractures permanently remove stress from the cords, myofibroblast apoptosis ensues. This marks the final involutional and static stage of the disease.[1]

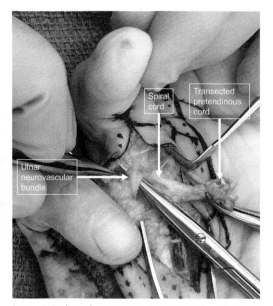

Fig. 1. Spiral cord traversing deep to NV bundle. Note the resulting superficial and central displacement of the NV bundle. (*Courtesy of* Brian W. Starr, MD.)

As these contractures are allowed to persist, the flexed posture of the fingers results in anatomic changes of the surrounding anatomy. Chronic contractures may result in attenuation of the sagittal bands at the MCP joint, central slip disruption and resulting Boutonniere deformity at the PIP joint, or mallet finger deformities. Contracture of the surrounding soft tissues, including the collateral ligaments of the MCP and PIP joints as well as the NV structures, also occurs in longstanding DD.

EVALUATION

Signs of early DD are frequently underreported by patients and go unnoticed by health care providers. The right hand is more frequently affected than the left, with the ring finger being the most commonly affected digit.[18] Nodules are the first physical change noted by patients 60% of the time. These nodules are fixed to the overlying dermis and can be tender or itchy.[19] Garrod pads are dorsal Dupuytren nodules that present on the extensor surfaces of digital joints. These dorsal nodules often precede palmar manifestations of DD and may indicate a more aggressive biology of disease.[20] Longitudinal cords on the palmar aspect of the hand feel like a thickening of the underlying fascia that may only be appreciated on digital extension during early disease. It is common for patients to also have pitting of the palmar skin, representing contraction of the underlying dermis and adhesion to the pathologic cord.

The initial manifestation of DC presents as a restriction in passive extension, typically caused by a contracted cord impacting the MCP and PIP joints of the fingers. Nearly all these cords can be felt through fingertip pressure. Given that nonnodular cords are soft when the fingers are in a position of rest but become firm when under tension, the clinician discerns contracted cords while the patient's finger is moved passively from a flexed to an extended position. These cords typically form along identifiable lines of mechanical tension generated by either passive extension or abduction.

In a study looking at DD progression, patients who initially presented with nodules would progress to DC only 10% of the time at an average of 9 year follow-up. Forty percentage of patients had progressed to a cord without contracture, and 40% stayed the same.[21] A separate study demonstrated that 66% of patients presenting with nodules or cords without contracture would not progress to contracture over an 18 year follow-up.[22] Due to the differential diagnosis, including less common tumors, these patients should be seen at scheduled follow-up intervals in order to ensure the masses do not undergo any significant changes.

THERAPEUTIC OPTIONS
General Indications

All existing DC interventions are palliative and prone to recurrence. The literature has yet to delineate an optimal time for intervention that would yield the best outcomes. Thorough discussion with the patient should elucidate any issues concerning their functional status, including difficulty with facial hygiene, the inability to lay the hand flap on a table (the tabletop test), and the inability to place one's hand into a pant pocket (the pocket test). Interventions should generally be undertaken before the severity of the contracture reaches approximately 35° to 40° at the PIP joint.[17]

Nodules

In general, isolated nodules are not an indication for surgical intervention. Approximately half of all patients with nodules will go on to develop cords, and only a small percentage of these patients ultimately undergo surgical intervention.[21] A nonrandomized case series assessed injection of triamcinolone acetonide into 75 patients with palmar nodules. After an average of 3.2 injections per nodule, 97% of the hands showed regression of disease as exhibited by a softening or flattening of the nodule. Although a few patients did not experience recurrence or reactivation of the disease in the injected nodules or development of new nodules, 50% of patients did experience reactivation of disease in the nodules 1 to 3 years after the last injection, necessitating 1 or more injections.[23]

Minimally Invasive Techniques

Percutaneous needle fasciotomy
Percutaneous needle fasciotomy (PNF) was first described by Sir Astley Cooper in 1822 and later popularized by Dr Jean-Luc Lermusiaux in France.[24] The indications for the procedure are not very well defined. At a minimum, the patient must be cooperative for an awake procedure with a palpable tensionable cord. Despite its minimally invasive nature, PNF is not without risk. Skin rupture, infection, digital nerve division, flexor tendon rupture, and false aneurysm have all been reported as complications associated with the procedure.[25] Contraindications include lack of a palpable cord, rapid recurrence in a young patient, wounds, or infection in the area of the procedure, and postsurgical digital recurrences.

The technique is classically described as being performed in a distal to proximal direction. The portals for needle entry are anesthetized with a small amount of local anesthetic intradermally so as to avoid anesthetizing the underlying digital nerves. A small hypodermic needle is then used in small puncture maneuvers to repeatedly weaken the cord while it is held on tension. Ultimately, an extension maneuver is performed on the finger to achieve rupture of the cord and joint extension.

Studies have demonstrated the cost-effectiveness of PNF over other techniques. Recurrence rates seem to vary depending on the extent of disease at intervention, at about 10% per year and 50% at 5 years.[26] More severe deformities do not have as significant a correction, and the results decrease more rapidly over time.[1,27] However, satisfaction scores for the procedure are very high, and the majority of patients would recommend the procedure or undergo PNF again.[28]

Enzymatic fasciotomy
The Food and Drug Administration approved the collagenase Clostridium histolyticum (CCH) for the management of DD in 2010. It is contraindicated in patients who are allergic to collagenase, and the safety profile is unknown in patients who are pregnant or breast feeding. The technique involves injection into the substance of the pathologic cords with a small amount of CCH in 3 closely spaced locations along the cord. After 1 to 4 days, the patient returns to clinic for extension manipulation of the finger with cord rupture.

Similar to PNF, patients with joint contractures of less than 50° of the MCP and less than 40° of the PIP have better overall response and results to CCH injection.[29,30] Complication rates demonstrate a very low incidence of neuropraxia (4.4%), complex regional pain syndrome (0.1%), and tendon injury (0.3%).[31] Cost analysis studies demonstrate that CCH injection is a cost-effective alternative to open fasciectomy with a shortened return to work or daily activity.[32]

Surgical fasciectomy
Open surgical fasciectomy includes 3 distinct approaches: segmental, regional, and radical. Segmental fasciectomy involves removing small segments of the diseased cords with only minimal dissection to allow for full extension of the finger. Regional fasciectomy involves excision of all diseased tissue. Radical fasciectomy refers to removal of the entirety of the palmar fascia and the surrounding subcutaneous tissue. Radical fasciectomy is no longer performed, as it carries significant morbidity without additional benefit.

Segmental fasciectomy is performed through multiple small incisions along the affected area. Only pathology centered over these incisions is excised, and the skin is closed primarily. Regional fasciectomy, on the other hand, requires forethought of incision placement. Primary longitudinal or zig-zag incisions are designed over the fingers that converge in the palm in order to address multiple fingers. Local flaps such as Z plasty as well as V-Y flaps should be planned prior to making skin incisions in anticipation of the potential for having tight or insufficient skin to close the wounds. Studies have shown that the addition of small skin grafts to small areas of open wounds do not improve early outcomes or later recurrence rates (Fig. 2).[33] As originally described by McCash, a modified version that leaves palmar incisions open in order to close more distal incisions has good functional results, appropriate healing, and high patient satisfaction.[34]

Since open fasciectomy requires the use of an operating room and an anesthesia team, it is not as cost-effective as PNF. However, using the definition of recurrence as the presence of 20° of contracture more at 1 year compared to the amount of contracture present at 6 weeks postoperatively, recurrence rates for open fasciectomy have been recorded as low as 5%.[35] It is clear in the literature that recurrence rates for open fasciectomy are lower than those of both PNF and injection of CCH. **Figs. 2–7** demonstrate a classic presentation of bilateral DD, including early and late postoperative outcomes and contralateral disease progression.

Postfasciectomy flare reaction (PFFR) is defined as prolonged swelling, pain, and stiffness following DC palmar fasciectomy, with more extensive dissections leading to greater symptoms. The incidence of PFFR is approximately 10%. This can continue for months after surgery and may lead to permanent stiffness in 5% of patients.[36] Digital nerve injury is perhaps the most well-known and feared complication of surgical intervention. The literature cites a 3% incidence of nerve injury during palmar fasciectomy, and a 15% risk of injury in cases of recurrent DC undergoing repeat fasciectomy.[36]

Skeletal traction

Treatment of severe PIP joint contracture greater than 60° adds additional complication to the paradigm. After such extensive joint contracture has taken place, many surrounding structures have undergone changes in length that require attention. The extensor mechanism tends to stretch out over the PIP joint, leading to laxity and imbalance.

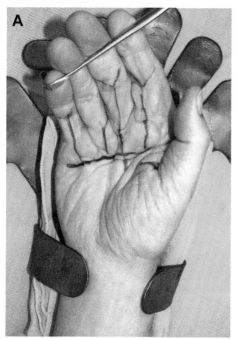 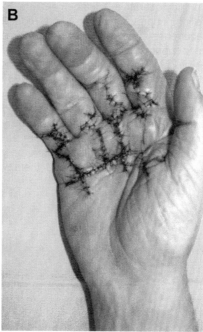

Fig. 2. A 55 year old gentleman with advanced DCs of all digits of the right hand. (*A*) Our preferred incision design includes a V extension at the level of the PIP joint. (*B*) Initial exposure includes a straight longitudinal incision; however, we routinely perform a 60° Z-plasty at the base of the finger, prior to closure. (*Courtesy of* Kevin C. Chung, MD.)

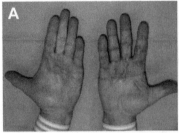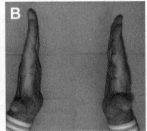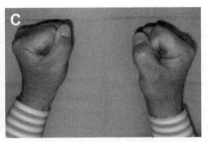

Fig. 3. (*A–C*) Two months postop limited fasciectomy of the right thumb, index, middle, ring, and small fingers. Please note that this patient has worked diligently with hand therapy and demonstrates a remarkably swift recovery. It is not uncommon for patients to have persistent swelling and range of motion deficits several months following surgery. (*Courtesy of* Kevin C. Chung, MD).

Collateral ligaments around the joint have shortened and tightened, NV structures have shortened due to their constant flexion posture, and the skin has undergone contracture as well. Addressing these issues adequately necessitates a staged approach.[37]

Application of an external skeletal traction device allows the soft tissues surrounding the PIP joint to stretch to the point of allowing further surgical intervention to take place. The Boutonniere deformity associated with PIP flexion contracture is best treated with PIP fusion, although other options such as skeletal shortening, middle phalangectomy, and amputation remain more invasive options.[38]

POSTOPERATIVE MANAGEMENT

The goals of postoperative management are to reduce swelling, improve function, and reduce long-term recurrence rates. There is no good clinical literature to support any particular form of postoperative protocol. The evidence to support postoperative splinting is equivocal, with one study demonstrating marginally decreased finger flexion due to immobilization.[39] A separate study showed no differences in self-reported upper limb disability or active range of motion between a group of patients who were all routinely splinted after surgery and a group of patients receiving hand therapy

and only splinted if and when contractures occurred.[40] The current trend with certified hand therapists is toward intermittent compression for management of edema along with active motion.

FUTURE

Future directions and consideration for the treatment of DD involve much earlier detection of the disease process. As DD is a systemic medical condition, identification of gene loci within the genome that predispose patients to the disease will help with earlier detection of disease. The implementation of machine learning algorithms and quantum computing, which are in their nascency, will undoubtably assist in this endeavor. Likely, a treatment paradigm paralleling the course of disease-modifying antirheumatologic agents will be a spoke in the wheel of treatment options in the future.

EDITORS' COMMENTARY (IN LIEU OF SUMMARY SECTION)

There is no shortage of debate surrounding the optimal treatment of DD. Surgeons across specialties, regions, cultures, and health care systems are likely to each have a nuanced approach to care. Differences aside, one core tenet of Dupuytren

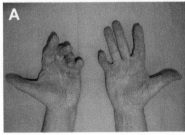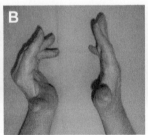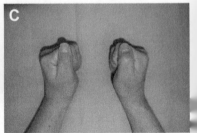

Fig. 4. (*A–C*) Four and a half years postop limited fasciectomy of the right thumb, index, middle, ring, and small fingers. Note the recurrence of right-sided contractures involving the small and index fingers. The previously asymptomatic cords of the left hand have progressed to debilitating contractures. (*Courtesy of* Kevin C. Chung, MD).

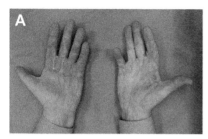
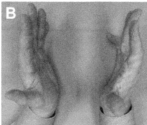
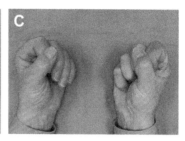

Fig. 5. (*A–C*) Two months postop left index, middle, ring, and small finger limited fasciectomy. (*Courtesy of* Kevin C. Chung, MD.)

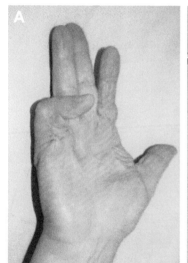
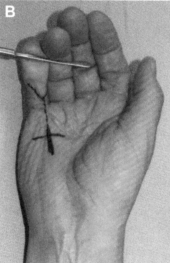
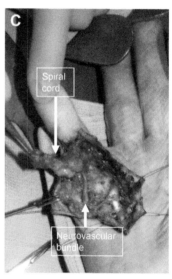

Fig. 6. (*A–C*) Now 6 years postop right-sided fasciectomy, the right small finger demonstrates a recurrent contracture with a 60°PIPJ contracture. The small finger often frustrates patients and surgeons, as it is especially prone to recurrence. Contractures of this digit pose problems with routine facial hygiene and with placing a hand in a pocket. (*A*) Preop contracture. (*B*) Incision design. (*C*) Excision of recurrent spiral cord and PIP joint capsulotomy. (*Courtesy of* Kevin C. Chung, MD.)

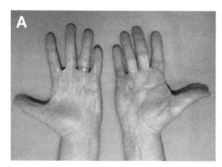
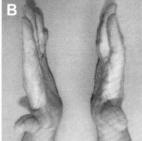
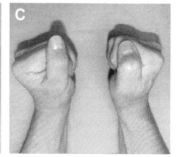

Fig. 7. (*A–C*) Superb functional result 1 month postop right small finger fasciectomy and PIP joint capsulotomy. (*Courtesy of* Kevin C. Chung, MD.)

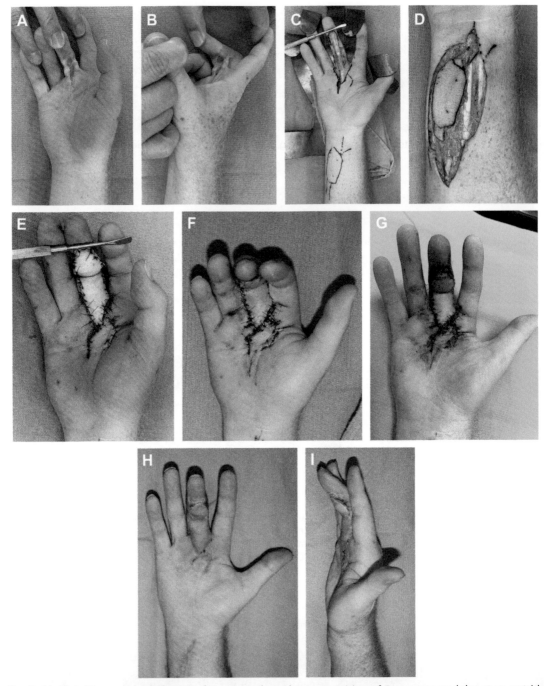

Fig. 8. (*A, B*) A 45 year old gentleman who previously underwent excision of Dupuytren nodules at an outside facility. He subsequently developed an accelerated progression of DC and hypertrophic scarring with a 90° PIP joint contracture. (*C, D*) In our experience, these complex cases are best managed with an arterialized venous flow through flap. (*C*) Complete, dermofascial excision of diseased tissue and marking of venous flow through flap proximally. (*D*) Venous flap incised with centrally located proximal and distal veins preserved. (*E–G*) Typical progression of color in a venous flow through scenario. (*E*) Intraop appearance. (*F*) Three days postop. (*G*) Ten days postop. (*H, I*) One month postop. (*Courtesy of* Kevin C. Chung, MD.)

treatment is a patient-centered approach that is guided by shared decision-making. In our practices—high-volume academic medical centers in the mid-western United States—we frequently see patients with advanced, debilitating disease that affects the PIP joint. These patients are no longer ideal candidates for nonsurgical treatment. However, patients who present with mild disease (PIP joint contracture <30°) that does not interfere with daily life, warrant careful consideration. Thorough patient counseling is essential, not only to discuss risks, benefits, and alternatives—*including observation alone*—but also to calibrate patient expectations.

Needle aponeurotomy and collagenase injection are important, minimally invasive treatment options for select patients. The ideal candidate presents with a palpable, distinct cord in the palm, with an isolated MCP joint contracture. A contracture that also affects the PIP joint is not an absolute contraindication; however, patients must be counseled that postintervention residual PIP joint deformity is not uncommon. In the properly selected patient, either needle fenestration or collagenase injection can be very satisfying for both patient and surgeon. Though historical literature is mixed and has pointed to similar efficacy and recurrence rates, one recent randomized controlled trial demonstrated a statistically significant lower rate of recurrence at 3 years in patients with isolated MCP joint contractures treated with collagenase as opposed to needle aponeurotomy.[41] This contrasts with the large retrospective review from Leafblad and colleagues that noted that collagenase treatment was associated with a higher rate of reintervention at 2 years (41% vs 4%) but a comparable rate of reintervention at years (55% vs 61%).[42]

In our practice, patients with severe disease, with multiple cords affecting the PIP, are candidates for surgical intervention. The surgeon must have a clear understanding of normal and pathologic anatomy and should be able to anticipate the location of displaced NV structures. Though rare (2%–3%), the risk for inadvertent injury to NV structures should be explicitly discussed with the patient preoperatively. This risk increases 10 fold in cases requiring reoperation. Patients must also be aware of other untoward events, including wound healing complications, hematoma, incision site pain, complex regional pain syndrome, and early recurrence. Though not a complication per se, long-lasting edema and stiffness are common postoperatively. prospective cohort study found a persistent loss active finger flexion during the first year following surgery.[43]

Our preferred surgical technique is delineated in the prior in-text figures. A longitudinal approach to the digit with a V extension provides an excellent exposure and permits Z-lengthening prior to closure. In experienced hands, flap elevation and dissection are best performed with a knife, using a "push" technique. Blunt dissection using scissors risks more extensive soft tissue trauma and potential for neuropraxia and vessel contusion. NV bundles should be identified in the "soft spot" at the level of the PIP joint. The bundle is most superficial in this location and should be visualized and protected prior to cord removal. If PIP joint contracture persists following removal of all cords, a volar capsulotomy is performed. The A3 pulley is incised and the flexor tendons are retracted to either side to expose the volar plate. The proximal volar plate is then released, extending to the volar aspect of either collateral ligament. We routinely lengthen our closure with 60°degree Z-plasties made at the base of the digit. Permanent sutures are removed at 2 weeks. Hand therapy is initiated immediately postoperatively. Night-time extension splinting is advised for the first 6 months.

In the case of aggressive and/or recurrent disease (ie, Dupuytren diathesis), when the skin is a limiting factor, the arterialized venous flow through flap can offer a versatile solution. Flaps designed along the distal volar forearm are thin and versatile, with vessels with excellent caliber match to the digital vessels. Unlike conventional flaps, flap veins and the venous plexus are solely responsible for inflow and outflow in venous flow-through flaps. Surgeons should be mindful that because of this the postoperative flap appearance varies substantially compared to traditional flaps (**Fig. 8**).

CLINICS CARE POINTS

- In choosing among several treatment options, patient and surgeon benefit from a patient-centered approach that is guided by shared decision-making.

- The ideal candidate for needle aponeurotomy or collagenase injection presents with a palpable, distinct cord in the palm, with an isolated MCP joint contracture. Five-year recurrence of either approach is upwards of 50%.

- In our practice, patients with severe disease, with multiple cords affecting the PIP, are candidates for open fasciectomy.

- Surgical dissection is best performed sharply, with a knife, taking care to identify NV structures in predictable locations prior to excising cords.

DISCLOSURE

The authors have nothing to disclose.

REFERENCES

1. S 'Pederson W, Hotchkiss R, Kozin S, Cohen M. 7th edition. Green's operative hand surgery, vol. 1. Berkeley, CA: Elsevier; 2017.
2. Tubiana R. Dupuytren's disease of the radial side of the hand. Hand Clin 1999;15(1):149–59.
3. Lanting R, Broekstra DC, Werker PMN, et al. A systematic review and meta-analysis on the prevalence of Dupuytren disease in the general population of Western countries. Plast Reconstr Surg 2014; 133(3):593–603.
4. Lanting R, van den Heuvel ER, Westerink B, et al. Prevalence of dupuytren disease in The Netherlands. Plast Reconstr Surg 2013;132(2): 394–403.
5. Hu FZ, Nystrom A, Ahmed A, et al. Mapping of an autosomal dominant gene for Dupuytren's contracture to chromosome 16q in a Swedish family. Clin Genet 2005;68(5):424–9.
6. Saboeiro AP, Porkorny JJ, Shehadi SI, et al. Racial distribution of dupuytren's disease in department of veterans affairs patients. Plast Reconstr Surg 2000;106(1):71–5.
7. Zemel NP. Dupuytren's contracture in women. Hand Clin 1991;7(4):707–11. discussion 713.
8. Becker K, Tinschert S, Lienert A, et al. The importance of genetic susceptibility in Dupuytren's disease. Clin Genet 2015;87(5):483–7.
9. Dolmans GH, Werker PM, Hennies HC, et al. Wnt signaling and Dupuytren's disease. N Engl J Med 2011;365(4):307–17.
10. Nyberg LM, Bias WB, Hochberg MC, et al. Identification of an inherited form of Peyronie's disease with autosomal dominant inheritance and association with Dupuytren's contracture and histocompatibility B7 cross-reacting antigens. J Urol 1982; 128(1):48–51.
11. Brickley-Parsons D, Glimcher MJ, Smith RJ, et al. Biochemical changes in the collagen of the palmar fascia in patients with Dupuytren's disease. J Bone Joint Surg Am 1981;63(5):787–97.
12. Maccallum P, Hueston JT. The pathology of Dupuytren's contracture. Aust N Z J Surg 1962;31:241–53.
13. Fraser Leversedge, Charles Goldfarb, Martin Boyer. A Pocketbook Manual of Hand and Upper Extremity Anatomy.; 2010.
14. White S. Anatomy of the palmar fascia on the ulnar border of the hand. J Hand Surg Br 1984;9(1):50–6.
15. McFarlane RM. Patterns of the diseased fascia in the fingers in Dupuytren's contracture. Displacement of the neurovascular bundle. Plast Reconstr Surg 1974;54(1):31–44.
16. Umlas ME, Bischoff RJ, Gelberman RH. Predictors of neurovascular displacement in hands with Dupuytren's contracture. J Hand Surg Br 1994;19(5): 664–6.
17. Trickett RW, Savage R, Logan AJ. Angular correction related to excision of specific cords in fasciectomy for Dupuytren's disease. J Hand Surg Eur 2014; 39(5):472–6.
18. BOYES JH. Dupuytren's contracture; notes on the age at onset and the relationship to handedness. Am J Surg 1954;88(1):147–54.
19. Dibenedetti DB, Nguyen D, Zografos L, et al. Prevalence, incidence, and treatments of Dupuytren's disease in the United States: results from a population-based study. Hand (N Y) 2011;6(2):149–58.
20. Hueston JT. Some observations on knuckle pads. J Hand Surg Br 1984;9(1):75–8.
21. Reilly RM, Stern PJ, Goldfarb CA. A retrospective review of the management of Dupuytren's nodules. J Hand Surg Am 2005;30(5):1014–8.
22. Gudmundsson KG, Arngrimsson R, Jónsson T. Eighteen years follow-up study of the clinical manifestations and progression of Dupuytren's disease. Scand J Rheumatol 2001;30(1):31–4.
23. Ketchum LD, Donahue TK. The injection of nodules of Dupuytren's disease with triamcinolone acetonide. J Hand Surg Am 2000;25(6):1157–62.
24. Foucher G, Medina J, Navarro R. Percutaneous needle aponeurotomy: complications and results. J Hand Surg Br 2003;28(5):427–31.
25. Symes T, Stothard J. Two significant complications following percutaneous needle fasciotomy in a patient on anticoagulants. J Hand Surg Br 2006; 31(6):606–7.
26. Badois FJ, Lermusiaux JL, Massé C, et al. [Non-surgical treatment of Dupuytren disease using needle fasciotomy]. Rev Rhum Ed Fr 1993;60(11):808–13.
27. Pereira A, Massada M, Sousa R, et al. Percutaneous needle fasciotomy in Dupuytren's contracture: is it a viable technique? Acta Orthop Belg 2012;78(1): 30–4.
28. Toppi JT, Trompf L, Smoll NR, et al. Dupuytren's contracture: an analysis of outcomes of percutaneous needle fasciotomy versus open fasciectomy. ANZ J Surg 2015;85(9):639–43.
29. Hurst LC, Badalamente MA, Hentz VR, et al. Injectable collagenase clostridium histolyticum for Dupuytren's contracture. N Engl J Med 2009;361(10): 968–79.
30. Gilpin D, Coleman S, Hall S, et al. Injectable collagenase Clostridium histolyticum: a new nonsurgical treatment for Dupuytren's disease. J Hand Surg Am 2010;35(12):2027–20238.e1.
31. Smeraglia F, Del Buono A, Maffulli N. Collagenase clostridium histolyticum in Dupuytren's contracture: a systematic review. Br Med Bull 2016;118(1): 149–58.

32. Naam NH. Functional outcome of collagenase injections compared with fasciectomy in treatment of Dupuytren's contracture. Hand (N Y) 2013;8(4):410–6.

33. Ullah AS, Dias JJ, Bhowal B. Does a "firebreak" full-thickness skin graft prevent recurrence after surgery for Dupuytren's contracture?: a prospective, randomised trial. J Bone Joint Surg Br 2009;91(3):374–8.

34. Lesiak AC, Jarrett NJ, Imbriglia JE. Modified McCash technique for management of dupuytren contracture. J Hand Surg Am 2017;42(5):395.e1–5.

35. Radhamony NG, Nair RR, Sreenivasan S, et al. Residual deformity versus recurrence following Dupuytren's palmar fasciectomy-a long term follow-up of 142 cases. Ann Med Surg (Lond) 2022;73:103224.

36. Denkler K. Surgical complications associated with fasciectomy for dupuytren's disease: a 20-year review of the English literature. Eplasty 2010;10:e15.

37. Craft RO, Smith AA, Coakley B, et al. Preliminary soft-tissue distraction versus checkrein ligament release after fasciectomy in the treatment of dupuytren proximal interphalangeal joint contractures. Plast Reconstr Surg 2011;128(5):1107–13.

38. Eiriksdottir A, Atroshi I. A new finger-preserving procedure as an alternative to amputation in recurrent severe Dupuytren contracture of the small finger. BMC Musculoskelet Disord 2019;20(1):323.

39. Kemler MA, Houpt P, van der Horst CMAM. A pilot study assessing the effectiveness of postoperative splinting after limited fasciectomy for Dupuytren's disease. J Hand Surg Eur 2012;37(8):733–7.

40. Jerosch-Herold C, Shepstone L, Chojnowski AJ, et al. Night-time splinting after fasciectomy or dermo-fasciectomy for Dupuytren's contracture: a pragmatic, multi-centre, randomised controlled trial. BMC Musculoskelet Disord 2011;12:136.

41. Jørgensen RW, Jensen CH, Jørring S. Three-year recurrence of dupuytren contracture after needle fasciotomy or collagenase injection: a randomized controlled trial. Plast Reconstr Surg 2023 Feb 1;151(2):365–71.

42. Leafblad ND, Wagner E, Wanderman NR, et al. Outcomes and direct costs of needle aponeurotomy, collagenase injection, and fasciectomy in the treatment of dupuytren contracture. J Hand Surg Am 2019 Nov;44(11):919–27.

43. Engstrand C, Krevers B, Nylander G, et al. Hand function and quality of life before and after fasciectomy for Dupuytren contracture. J Hand Surg Am 2014 Jul;39(7):1333–43.e2.

Optimizing Outcomes in the Management of the Burned Hand

Elizabeth Dale Slater, MD*, Andrew Joseph James, BS, John Bradford Hill, MD

KEYWORDS

• Hand burn • Acute management • Chronic management • Hand burn deformity • Hand surgery

KEY POINTS

• Hand burns are highly morbid and common in severe burn patients.
• Appropriate acute intervention plays a key role in preventing downstream complications, and may require pinning, dermal matrices, and/or flap coverage.
• Burn deformity correction and scar care include fundamental local flaps, free flaps, and laser therapy.

INTRODUCTION

The hand is involved in 80% of all severe burn injuries.[1] Each hand accounts for only 3% of the total body surface area (TBSA) but injury to this small area is associated with significant physical disability and psychological distress.[2] We use our hands for tactile interaction with the world around us, activities of daily living, and functional independence, and as such, they are an early treatment priority. Here, the authors present a comprehensive approach to treatment of the burned hand, including considerations for acute management, reconstruction, and key complications that may arise.

DISCUSSION

Escharotomy and Compartment Release

Acute escharotomy and compartment release, especially in the forearms, hands, and digits (Fig. 1), are crucial. For full-thickness finger injuries with vascular compromise, a mid-lateral incision is recommended to alleviate pressure on neurovascular bundles.

Electrical burns require careful consideration due to the risk of deep injury in poorly conductive structures like bone and tendon. The severity of an electrical injury is determined by the flow of electric current through the body, as well as circuit voltage, tissue resistance, current amperage, current pathway, and duration of contact. When charged particles interact with tissue molecules, they release energy in the form of heat. The formula for electrical power, $E = I^2Rt$ (E = energy, I = current, R = resistance, t = time), describes the amount of heat dissipated by the electric current. Most tissue damage results from cell membrane disruption. Electrical injuries are typically categorized as either high voltage (>1000 V) or low voltage (<1000 V).[3]

Acute onset peripheral neuropathy is common in electrical injuries, especially high- voltage injuries, and warrants timely operative decompression.[4,5] In a review of burn unit admissions, Smith and colleagues found that 22% of electrical burn patients sustained permanent nerve injury.[6] Carpal tunnel syndrome has been identified as the most common compressive neuropathy in

Department of Plastic Surgery, Vanderbilt University Medical Center, 1161 21st Avenue South, Suite S-2221, Nashville, TN 37232, USA
* Corresponding author. Department of Plastic Surgery, Vanderbilt University Medical Center, 1161 21st Avenue South, Suite S-2221, Nashville, TN 37232.
E-mail address: elizabeth.d.slater@vumc.org

Clin Plastic Surg 51 (2024) 539–551
https://doi.org/10.1016/j.cps.2024.04.003
0094-1298/24/Published by Elsevier Inc.

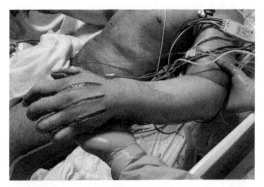

Fig. 1. Full thickness, circumferential hand and forearm burn treated in the acute setting with bedside digital, hand, and forearm escharotomies.

electrical and thermal burn patients.[7] Decompressive fasciotomies with carpal tunnel release are common practice in the setting of high-voltage electrical injuries; however, the evidence is mixed on whether this is necessary as a standard precaution.[8] The authors err on the side of caution; if there are symptoms of median nerve compression, urgent release is performed. In the intubated, sedated, or non-responsive patient, injury severe enough to cause regional necrosis, that is, circumferential eschar or substantial swelling at the wrist is an indication for carpal tunnel release. Patients are followed with serial examinations for several weeks and electrodiagnostic studies are a useful adjunct in patients with intact skin. In patients with open wounds, dedicated ultrasound can be used to better define areas of focal nerve compression or caliber changes.

Tangential Debridement

An understanding of burn mechanisms and injury progression guides effective debridement and coverage. Early excision and grafting are the current standard of care and is essential for optimal outcomes in hand burns. Tangential excision, often using a Weck-Goulian knife, is the preferred method. Debridement consists of meticulous layer-by-layer removal of non-viable tissue until healthy, bleeding tissue is encountered. Traditional early management involves blade excision to bleeding tissue but has been challenged by the promise of enzymatic debridement, showing potential for good post-operative hand function.[5,9] Additionally, hydro-dissection has been shown in several studies to decrease blood loss and inadvertent removal of healthy tissue.[10,11] However, this is most useful after 5 to 7 days when the eschar has begun to separate, and early excision typically make this unneccesary in our practice. Complete removal of devitalized tissue is crucial

to avoid hindering graft revascularization and prevent infection. Paratenon overlying extensor tendons should be preserved, whenever possible, to maintain a viable bed.

Positioning

To prevent downstream sequelae, the hand should be splinted or pinned in the intrinsic plus position as soon as possible after injury.[12] Intrinsic plus positioning involves full extension of the proximal interphalangeal (PIP) and distal interphalangeal (DIP) joints, 70° of flexion at the metacarpophalangeal (MCP) joints, and a 30° extension at the wrist. This posture can be maintained with a volar thermoplastic or plaster mold, or by pinning with Kirschner wires across the MCPs to facilitate prehension and interphalangeal flexion. The authors recommend pinning for improved reliability, as splinting requires significant oversight and patient compliance. This positioning reduces tension on the extensor apparatus after deep dorsal hand burns.[13] It also optimizes tension across the small joints of the hand, and prevents shortening of stabilizing ligaments and disruption of the delicate equilibrium between intrinsic and extrinsic muscles.[13,14] Splinting the elbow in full extension is favorable for vascular function, preservation of the joint, and preventing flexion contracture of the skin.[15] Elbow range of motion exercises should be incorporated early in treatment to ensure patients can flex the joint as elbow extension is not a position of function.

Regardless of graft fixation technique, early mobilization and formal hand therapy are critical to optimizing outcomes. The authors strongly advocate for manipulation of the hand joints under anesthesia whenever possible. If a patient has sedation administered for dressing changes, skin grafts, or other accessory procedures, this offers an opportunity to remove dressings and stretch the joints in a painless setting.

Management of Exposed Structures

Discussion of tendon exposure post-thermal injury must focus on differing treatments for the dorsal and volar aspects of the burned hand, as management significantly varies due to tissue heterogeneity. The dorsal hand has thin skin and is more susceptible to full-thickness thermal injury with exposure of underlying structures than the thicker palm of the hand. Fourth-degree injuries to the hand often result from contact, friction, or high voltage electrical injury.[16] Patient and injury characteristics guide management with the typical reconstructive ladder being skin grafting placement of a dermal substitute, or a flap-based reconstruction for increasingly severe injuries.

In these settings, immediate skin grafts are poorly adherent and often exhibit poor take because they rely on granulation tissue for local incorporation, and tendons are poorly vascularized beds.[17] Delaying dorsal skin grafting until granulation tissue covers the tendon enhances graft take, but also risks tendon desiccation and scar formation directly over the tendon apparatus.[18] Although not ideal, this approach may be suitable for patients with severe injuries who cannot tolerate a flap procedure or lack adequate donor skin.[19–22] In the authors practice, if sufficient skin is not available, artificial skin substitutes are placed initially with acceptable complication profiles, cosmesis, and functional outcomes.[21,22]

There are a myriad of dermal substitutes on the market.[23–26] In the acute setting, for patients with large TBSA burns, the authors favor Novosorb ™ biodegradable temporizing matrix (BTM) as first line as it is highly resistant to infection, and is often salvageable when infection is identified early. In addition, the outer silicone layer helps prevent insensible fluid losses and tissue desiccation.[27–29] However, it has poor integration over tendons. At times, the authors temporize with BTM, and when wounds are more stable in the periphery of the hand, the authors transition to Integra, which has a better take over tendons in the authors' experience. Notably, these tendons often require superficial debridement as the desiccated outer layers will not allow for incorporation of dermal matrices. Other promising new products include Matriderm[30] and Restrata,[31] but we do not have robust results to date with these. Notably, all dermal matrices require split-thickness grafts after incorporation but temporize and, in some instances, promote granulation for tendon coverage and protection.

For stable patients with good nutrition and operative candidacy, early flap coverage is a reliable option for dorsal hand wounds with exposure of tendon or bone. Ideally, tissue replacement in this setting would be heavily vascularized, thin, and allow the underlying tendons to glide comfortably. Local flaps including the posterior interosseous artery flap[32] and reverse radial forearm flap,[33] being moderately sized, avoid unnecessary bulk that could hinder motion during rehabilitation and have similar functional outcomes. In cases of substantial forearm injury, staged groin or abdominal flaps based on the epigastric circulation may be considered, although as traditionally described, they can result in excessive tissue bulk and require revision later.[34–37] The authors prefer a "superthin" version of the epigastric flaps for digit and

dorsal hand coverage (**Fig. 2**). Serratus anterior free flaps have been successfully utilized in this setting and represent a reliable option in patients with full-thickness dorsal injury.[38] For smaller digital burns, cross-finger flaps can be considered.[39] Venous flow-through flaps are also a reasonable choice and have been found to have robust microcirculation.[40,41] Flap choice is guided by donor site viability and the status of the patient. Those with burns affecting higher TBSAs may have limited options for both local pedicled flap and free flap reconstruction. Skin flaps may offer greater versatility for future elevation but often require subsequent soft tissue debulking. Muscle flaps will atrophy and thin over time; however, they are technically more challenging for future elevation when staged procedures such as skeletal, tendon reconstruction or tenolysis are anticipated.

SKIN GRAFTING
Dorsal Hand

Achieving durable dorsal hand coverage can be challenging. Superficial partial-thickness burns can be managed with immediate mobilization, wound care, and skin substitutes, such as Suprathel™, secured with sutures or fibrin sealant.[42–44] Suprathel™ is a synthetic bioabsorbable material that was engineered to mimic native epidermis and helps retain moisture to help prevent insensible losses.[43] For deep partial-thickness burns, debridement, whether surgical or enzymatic, prepares a wound bed for the application of skin substitutes, described earlier. For this mid-depth injury, the authors favor Suprathel™ or BTM (Novosorb) in the acute phase.[13,45]

For full-thickness injury, autologous skin grafting is an integral part of burn care, and thoughtful consideration must be used when grafting the highly mobile hand. As a general principle, grafts should be secured with the hand in a position that places maximal stretch on the grafted area. This aims to enhance mobility and reduce the detrimental effects of graft contracture during healing. Staging may be necessary, depending on the affected hand region. For instance, a patient with burns on both the dorsal and volar sides of a finger may require flexed positioning for dorsal coverage and extended positioning for volar coverage. Some advocate securing a skin graft with fibrin glue or sutures, enabling gentle range of motion (ROM) exercises on the first postoperative day. Others immobilize the fingers in the intrinsic-plus position using pins or K-wires for 6 weeks. A third group compromises between the two, recommending short-term splinting following graft placement.[42,46,47] The strategy

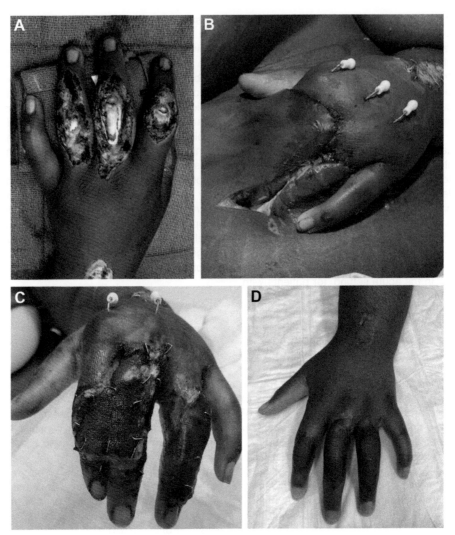

Fig. 2. Full thickness dorsal friction burn with exposed proximal interphalangeal joint and destruction of extensor mechanism. (*A*) Following debridement (*B*) digits pinned in extension and coverage with super-thin abdominal flap (*C*) following flap division and (*D*) release of syndactylized digits.

employed by the authors is to graft the dorsum of the hand in a flexed position to maximize the area of the skin paddle and to shape the graft to fit the 3-dimensional architecture of the web spaces.[48]

Initial coverage of the burned hand should use split-thickness grafts (**Fig. 3**). The standard depth for split-thickness grafts is 0.012 inches; however, thicker grafts offer better pliability and are used when available. This can require a "graft back" technique, whereby a graft harvest at 0.024 inch is placed on the hand and then a thin (0.010 inch) meshed graft is placed on the original donor site as a 0.024 inch donor site is nearly full thickness and will not heal by secondary intention. Alternatively, for patients with very large TBSA burns, harvesting a thinner graft is necessary due to the need to re-harvest from

the same site. In these instances, the authors will often harvest as thin as 0.010 inches, and use Recell™ to spray the donor site to ensure rapid healing for grafting remaining open wounds.[49]

While sheet grafts reduce the risk of contracture, they carry a higher risk of underlying hematoma or seroma, hindering graft take in small areas. In the authors practice, a dressing take-down on all hands with sheet grafts is performed on the first postoperative day to sharply open any fluid-filled raised areas, known as "blebs." This process, referred to as "deblebbing," helps prevent contamination issues and improves graft take. A follow-up check is conducted on the second postoperative day if a significant number of blebs were observed on the first day.[50]

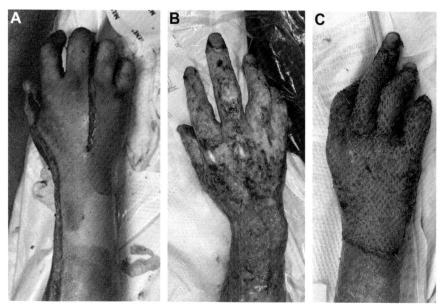

Fig. 3. Acute management of a severe dorsal hand burn (*A*) escharotomy (*B*) debridement (*C*) coverage with meshed split-thickness skin grafts.

In extensive burn injuries (50% TBSA and above), where unmeshed grafts may not be feasible, meshed grafts offer advantages in optimizing take (reduces seroma risk) and smaller donor sites are required.[50,51] Meshing, up to a maximum ratio of 1.5:1, reduces infection risk but is linked to higher contraction rates and undesirable cosmesis.[19] Meshing in the authors' institution is reserved for patients with high TBSA burns and limited donor sites. The dorsal hand is uniquely visible and mobile, and mesh ratios greater than 1.5:1 lead to increased scar contracture and worse cosmesis.[20]

Web Spaces

Few high-quality studies exist regarding the acute management of the burned web space. The primary focus in the current literature is centered around chronic management.[52] The mainstay of treatment is to achieve durable skin coverage and address contractures with a secondary operation if they arise.[53–56] The authors advocate for an appreciation of the conical shape of the dorsal web, and insist on creating a deep V-shaped graft up to the apex of the web (parallel to the MPJ), and ending at the natural web. Optimally, they also advocate for placing graft seams at the apex of each joint (MPJ, PIPJ, and DIPJ) with the digits in a flexed position to maximize the dorsal surface area and break the graft lines that tend to otherwise require z-plasties later when placed at the medial and ulnar edges of the digit.[48] These interventions dovetail to create a close approximation of the loose draping and distensibility of the native web spaces and joints. The first web space should be grafted with the thumb abducted from the hand, with the head of the first metacarpal tilted volarly to maximize the stretch on the web space.

Palmar Hand

Thick skin texture and fibrous protection of the palmar fascia allow expectant management for many volar burns with good wound care. When thermal injury exposes flexor tendons, early coverage is dependent on extent of injury. Frequently, such hands are not salvageable as palmar burns of that depth can cause thrombosis of neurovascular bundles. However, when the location is limited due to a focal contact burn, for example, early coverage is important, and regional flaps are optimal. The authors favor reverse radial forearm flaps in this setting. For palm or volar finger grafting, choices include split-thickness skin grafts (STSG), full-thickness skin grafts (FTSG), and medium-thickness glabrous skin grafts (MTGSG). MTGSG offers a close color and texture match, bringing glabrous structures directly to the injury site, potentially enhancing sensation and functionality, but donor sites are limited so these are only reasonable in small burns.[57]

MANAGEMENT OF COMMON HAND BURN COMPLICATIONS
A Web Space Contracture and Creep

First webspace contractures frequently occur with fibrosis of the adductor and first dorsal interosseus muscles or direct injury to the proximal joint capsule.[58] Contraction in an adducted position is most common and limits motion about the trapeziometacarpal joint. The skin contractures can be released with traditional z-plasty techniques (**Fig. 4**), local flaps (**Fig. 5**), or skin grafts. Simultaneous release of fibrotic and contracted adductor or first dorsal interosseous muscle is essential to achieving a complete release.[52,58] A 2020 retrospective review of 57 burned hands by Greyson and colleagues found that z-plasty and other local flaps were the most commonly performed reconstructive procedures in the first web space and that they required fewer revision procedures than both full-thickness and split-thickness skin grafts.[59]

The senior author recommends contracture release with a 5-flap z-plasty, sometimes referred to as a "jumping man flap," because this reconstruction reliably supplies the most critical central skin paddle for coverage. When grafting is needed, this typically only requires small pinch grafting at the edges which is better tolerated than a central graft (**Fig. 6**).[60] Web space creep can be addressed with a similar flap strategy. The authors also suggest the 5-flap z-plasty for other interdigital webs as well since this can also allow for deepening through the V-Y central inset. Flap options should be tailored to the patient presentation. In cases where the dorsal thenar eminence or snuffbox have substantial scarring, 5-flap z-plasty may prove challenging due to thick tissue and difficult mobilization in the middle of the web-space. In such cases, a 4-flap z-plasty could be a better alternative.

Boutonniere Deformity

Boutonniere deformity is caused by incompetence or damage to the central slip of the extensor apparatus. This may happen from direct thermal injury, desiccation from prolonged exposure, or loss of balance from long-standing contracture.[61] The inciting injury to the central slip disrupts the delicate balance between intrinsic and extrinsic forces and causes the lateral bands to slide volar to the *proximal interphalangeal joint* (PIP) joint axis of rotation. This destroys the extensor-flexor counterpoint in the PIP joint, resulting in unopposed PIP joint flexion and DIP joint hyperextension. Early intervention aimed at restoring dorsal coverage is critical to prevent extensor tendon desiccation, rupture, and subsequent boutonniere deformity. It is important to distinguish boutonniere deformity from digital flexion contracture, where volar scar tissue and flexor tendon damage lead to flexion at both PIP and DIP joints (**Fig. 7**).

Surgical correction of chronic boutonniere deformity is challenging and often yields unsatisfactory outcomes. Options include ligamentous rearrangement, PIP joint arthrodesis, or amputation in the setting of significant disability. Soft tissue rearrangements face varying success due to local scarring and tension on the reconstruction from underlying tendinous interactions, leading to early or late breakdown. In chronic cases, the central slip is often absent or nonviable, necessitating surgeons to centralize lateral bands or use tendon grafts for functional anatomic reconstruction.[61] Unfortunately, chronic flexion deformities may cause shortening of neuromuscular structures and lead to vascular compromise when restored to an extended position.[61] In these instances, it is important to assess perfusion off tourniquet, and consider gradually allowing the fingers to extend when perfusion comes into question. Patient characteristics and local tissue viability play a key role in operative strategy. Extensive patient counseling and consideration must be undertaken for chronic boutonniere deformities in burn

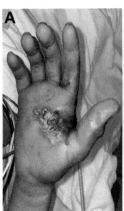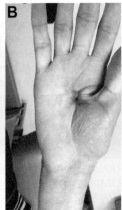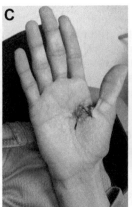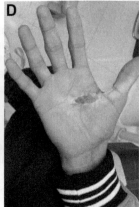

Fig. 4. Electrical injury to the hand resulting in first webspace adduction contracture. (*A*) Initial presentation (*B*) healed with conservative, non-operative treatment (*C, D*) adduction contracture treated with Z-plasty release.

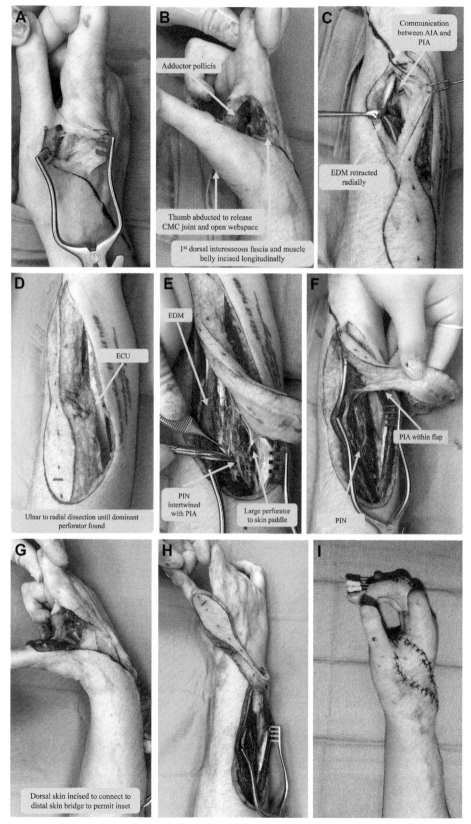

Fig. 5. Figures courtesy of Dr Chung. Severe first webspace/adduction contracture requiring release and flap resurfacing via PIA flap. (*A, B*) Release of first webspace (*C*) interval between ECU and EDM. (*D*) Perforator into skin paddle identified (*E*) septum raised from proximal to distal (*F*) PIA dissected free from PIN (*G*) dorsal skin incised (*H*) confirm adequate pedicle length (note dog ear is maintained) (*I*) flap inset/appearance 1-week post-op. ECU, extensor carpi ulnaris; EDM, extensor digiti minim; PIA, posterior interosseous artery; PIN, posterior interosseous nerve.

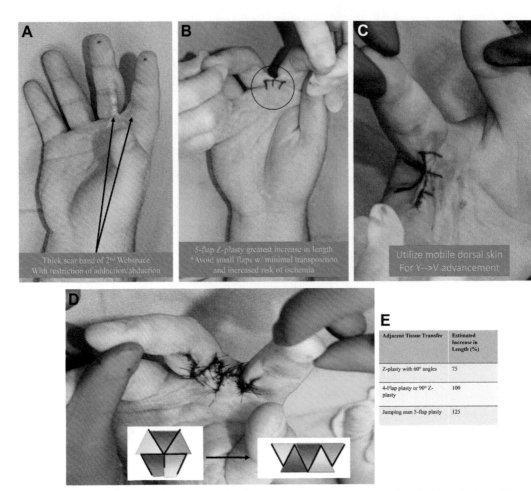

Fig. 6. Figures courtesy of Dr Chung. Second webspace scar contracture treated with 5-flap Z-plasty ("Jumping Man") technique. (*A*) Pre-opappearance demonstrating thick interdigital scar bands (*B, C*) Z-plasty design. (*D*) Flaps incised and inset. (*E*) Estimated length increase of common Z-plasty techniques.

patients to determine what—if any—surgical intervention may be appropriate, based on the extent of injury and the viability of surrounding tissue.

Flexion Contracture

Flexion contractures occur secondary to full-thickness injury to the palmar surface of the hand. Contact burns pose increased risk for full-thickness injury. If the protective palmar aponeurosis is breached by thermal injury, prompt evaluation is crucial, as infection and permanent disability are likely outcomes. Young children—who are ever-curious and explore their surroundings with their hands—are prone to severe palmar injuries from grasping hot objects and from the occasional treadmill friction burn. These injuries frequently require skin grafting, though there is a role for conservative management in a reliable patient with close follow-up. Nonoperative management should be forgone if injuries have not healed within 3 weeks. Adults are

more likely to sustain severe palmar burns via electrical injury. Most adult volar contact burns will heal spontaneously; however, electrical burns are often deeper than they appear. Nerves are particularly vulnerable and may require delayed reconstruction in patients with severe palmar electrical injury. [62]

Volar thermal injuries most commonly lead to burn cicatrix, graft contracture, or underlying flexor tendon damage, causing flexion in 1 or more digits.[63] These contractures are marked by fixed flexion at 1 or more IP joints or the MCP joint (see **Fig. 5**) and have variable treatment options based on structures involved.[63] Surgical treatment for more superficial injuries is routinely performed with z-plasty to the level of the tendon sheath. More complex soft tissue and joint injuries are mobilized based on the structures involved. In longstanding flexion contractures, volar plate, collateral, and checkrein ligaments may need to be released in sequential fashion. With release of severe flexion contractures, care must be taken to avoid placing

A

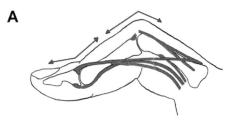

Boutonniere deformity with damaged central slip and extension at the distal interphalangeal joint

B

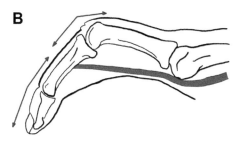

Flexion contracture with flexion at both interphalangeal joints

Fig. 7. Diagram of Boutonniere deformity (*A*) and flexion contracture (*B*) with emphasis on joint angles to clinically differentiate the two.

the neurovascular bundles in compromising traction.[61] In many ways, available joint and soft tissue options for this repair mirror those used in the treatment of Dupuytren's contracture, however, skin deficits and damage to other hand structures must be constant considerations and guide decision-making (see **Fig. 6**).

Extension Contracture

Extension contracture of the dorsal hand can be addressed with scar release and placement of an STSG with early motion to try to maintain tendon glide or with the pedicled and free flap reconstructive options mentioned in the Management of Exposed Structures section earlier. Extension contracture of a digit prevents finger flexion at 1 or more IP or MCP joints and usually presents with a finger that is partially flexed but cannot carry out active range of motion. A combination of both of these features creates the characteristic "claw" deformity, discussed later. Conservative interventions include manipulation under anesthesia, scar massage, laser therapy, and aggressive hand therapy. In severe contractures, or in cases of failed conservative management, surgical intervention may be indicated for optimal functional improvement. The surgeon should be prepared to release superficial skin and scar tissue, in addition to underlying joint capsular contracture and fibrosis.[61] In some instances, contracture release will recreate the soft tissue defect and warrant

resurfacing. The surgeon must be prepared to potentially address soft tissue deficits on the dorsum of the hand following contracture release.

Intrinsic Minus (Claw) Hand

Early mobilization and consultation with a dedicated hand therapist are crucial to enhance mobility and reduce the risk of debilitating contractures, particularly in deep burns affecting the dorsal hand.[64] If neglected, a severely burned hand is prone to develop intrinsic minus posture, characterized by hyperextension of the MCP joint and flexion of the PIP and DIP joints. This is induced by extrinsic muscle activation, accentuated by inadequate intrinsic counteraction due to significant hand swelling.[65] Over time, edema is replaced with fibrosis and scarring and leads to progressive deformity with MCP joint extension contracture and subluxation. Extensor tendons become scarred and adherent, and correction of the characteristic "claw hand" is no longer possible by conservative modalities. In patients with severe fibrosis, operative intervention targets release of the contracted dorsal MCP joint capsule, extensor tenolysis,[66] and temporary pinning in an effort to mobilize the joints and address intrinsic extensor tightness.[67] At the time of release, any exposed dorsal structures require prompt, durable coverage to prevent desiccation and additional morbidity.[67] Because most of the dorsal hand is previously injured in these settings, being prepared to provide flap coverage is critical. Sometimes a local flap like reverse radial forearm flap or posterior interosseus artery flap is available. If not, groin or epigastric flaps utilized as "superthin" flaps are the authors' preferred coverage (see **Fig. 2**).[36,37]

Digit Loss

Digit loss is an unfortunate outcome in hand burns but is sometimes unavoidable due to extensive damage. The decision to amputate considers damage to the flexor and extensor apparatus, neurovascular injury, and joint exposure. In cases of both flexor and extensor apparatus damage, transphalangeal or ray amputation may preserve hand function through removal of a minimally functional digit. While hand deformation can have psychosocial implications,[68] amputation of digits with fixed deformity can increase functionality (**Fig. 8**). However, the goal should generally be digit preservation, with particular emphasis on the thumb, as its absence can lead to up to a 40% reduction in hand functionality.[69] If the thumb has been compromised or lost, pollicization, metacarpal distraction osteogenesis lengthening, phalangealization, and toe transfers should be considered (See Chapter

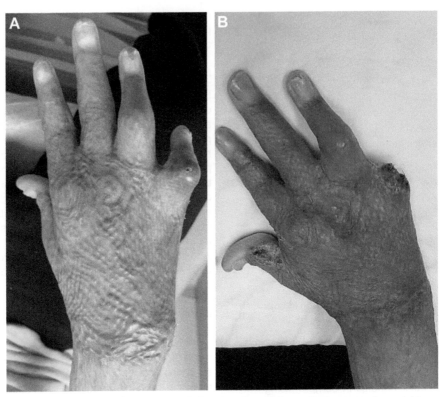

Fig. 8. Post-burn sequelae—Severe boutonniere deformity of small finger that was causing catching on clothing and causing functional impairment with facial hygiene. Note that the thumb and ring finger are also affected, but to a lesser extent. (*A*) Pre-op (*B*) post.amputation.

11—Preserving and Reconstructing the Traumatized Thumb).

Scar Rehabilitation

Burn scars cause both psychosocial distress and impair function in patients with extensive burns.[70] Scar therapy, including topical treatments and massage, remains a crucial aspect of treatment. Laser therapy has experienced a renaissance since the 1980s and is a versatile option for treatment of hypertrophic burn scars. The 2 primary laser therapies can be used concurrently as complementary treatments for enhanced effectiveness.

Pulsed dye laser (PDL) therapy uses a specific wavelength (typically 585–595 nm) to target and destroy superficial blood vessels formed during the healing of burn wounds. This approach aims to reduce local vascularity, improve color match, reduce pruritis, and induce rearrangement of the extracellular matrix by heating local collagen.[71] Ablative fractional resurfacing has deeper tissue penetration and creates a uniform grid of deep thermal injury which initiates collagen fibril production in a looser, more physiologic, orientation. This is accomplished using either a CO_2 or Erbium laser, and can assist with debulking, decreasing scar tension, and softening scars in preparation for revisionary procedures.[71]

SUMMARY

Proper acute management of burns leads to better long-term outcomes. Escharotomy or fasciotomy when indicated, coupled with adequate debridement, diligent hand positioning, and early rehabilitation are fundamental tenets. When deep structures are exposed, early durable soft tissue coverage is essential. Dermal substitutes, autologous skin grafting, and occasionally tissue transfer underly proper management schemes. When patients present with complex, chronic deformities, scar treatment and thorough releases lead to better secondary results.

CLINICS CARE POINTS

- Digital Escharotomy
  - Perform mid-lateral incision on the non-contact side for circumferential full-thickness finger burns with vascular compromise.

- Intrinsic Plus Positioning:
  - Keep PIP and DIP joints fully extended, MCP joints at 70° flexion, and wrist extended 30°.
  - Consider pinning the MCP joints into flexion.
- Dorsal Hand Burn Injuries:
  - Thin dorsal hand skin often leads to burn injuries reaching paratenon or tendon proper.
  - Address dorsal web conical shape with a deep V-shaped graft, placing seams at joint apexes.
- Web Space Contracture Release:
  - Utilize a 5-flap z-plasty ("jumping man flap") for reliable central skin paddle in most web space contractures.
- Chronic Boutonniere Deformity Correction:
  - Correct deformity through tendon rebalancing, PIP joint arthrodesis, or amputation for severe disability.
- Volar Thermal Injuries:
  - Flexion of digits may result from burn cicatrix, graft contracture, or underlying flexor tendon damage.
- Digit Loss in Hand Burns:
  - Unfortunate outcome sometimes unavoidable based on the extent of damage or lack of function.
- Laser Therapies for Scarring:
  - Pulsed dye and CO_2 fractional ablative lasers are primary options for addressing scarring in burns, often used concurrently.

DISCLOSURE

The authors have no financial relationships to disclose.

REFERENCES

1. Pensler JM, Steward R, Lewis SR, et al. Reconstruction of the burned palm: full-thickness versus split-thickness skin grafts–long-term follow-up. Plast Reconstr Surg 1988;81(1):46–9.
2. Grob M, Papadopulos NA, Zimmermann A, et al. The psychological impact of severe hand injury. J Hand Surg Eur 2008;33(3):358–62.
3. Prahlow JA, Ashraf Z, Plaza N, et al. Elevator-related deaths. J Forensic Sci 2020;65(3):823–32.
4. Strong AL, Agarwal S, Cederna PS, et al. Peripheral neuropathy and nerve compression syndromes in burns. Clin Plast Surg 2017;44(4):793–803.
5. Corrales-Benitez C, Gonzalez-Peinado D, Gonzalez-Miranda A, et al. Evaluation of burned hand function after enzymatic debridement. J Plast Reconstr Aesthetic Surg 2022;75(3):1048–56.
6. Harris RA, Iwamoto ET, Loh HH, et al. Site dependent analgesia after microinjection of morphine or lanthanum in rat brain. Proc West Pharmacol Soc 1975;18:275–8.
7. Ferguson JS, Franco J, Pollack J, et al. Compression neuropathy: a late finding in the postburn population: a four-year institutional review. J Burn Care Res May-Jun 2010;31(3):458–61.
8. Piccolo NS, Piccolo MS, Piccolo PD, et al. Escharotomies, fasciotomies and carpal tunnel release in burn patients–review of the literature and presentation of an algorithm for surgical decision making. Handchir Mikrochir Plast Chir 2007;39(3):161–7.
9. Hirche C, Kreken Almeland S, Dheansa B, et al. Eschar removal by bromelain based enzymatic debridement (Nexobrid(R)) in burns: European consensus guidelines update. Burns 2020;46(4): 782–96.
10. Kakagia DD, Karadimas EJ. The efficacy of versajet hydrosurgery system in burn surgery. a systematic review. J Burn Care Res 2018;39(2):188–200.
11. Klein MB, Hunter S, Heimbach DM, et al. The Versajet water dissector: a new tool for tangential excision. J Burn Care Rehabil Nov-Dec 2005;26(6): 483–7.
12. Kowalske KJ. Hand burns. Phys Med Rehabil Clin N Am 2011;22(2):249–59, vi.
13. Serror K, Chaouat M, Chatelain S, et al. External fixation during the acute phase of deep burned hands: description of saint louis' burn center technique. J Burn Care Res 2020;41(3):700–4.
14. James JI. The assessment and management of the injured hand. Hand 1970;2(2):97–105.
15. Procter F. Rehabilitation of the burn patient. Indian J Plast Surg 2010;43(Suppl):S101–13.
16. Hentz VR. Burns of the hand. Thermal, chemical, and electrical. Emerg Med Clin North Am 1985; 3(2):391–403.
17. Um JH, Jo DI, Kim SH. New proposal for skin grafts on tendon-exposed wounds. Arch Plast Surg 2022; 49(1):86–90.
18. Graham DJ, Clitherow HDS, Singh HP, et al. The effect of extensor tendon adhesions on finger motion. J Hand Surg Am 2019;44(10):903 e1–e903 e5.
19. Petry JJ, Wortham KA. Contraction and growth of wounds covered by meshed and non-meshed split thickness skin grafts. Br J Plast Surg 1986;39(4): 478–82.
20. Smith MA, Munster AM, Spence RJ. Burns of the hand and upper limb–a review. Burns 1998;24(6): 493–505.
21. Danin A, Georgesco G, Touze AL, et al. Assessment of burned hands reconstructed with Integra((R)) by

ultrasonography and elastometry. Burns 2012;38(7): 998–1004.

22. Dantzer E, Queruel P, Salinier L, et al. Dermal regeneration template for deep hand burns: clinical utility for both early grafting and reconstructive surgery. Br J Plast Surg 2003;56(8):764–74.

23. Yannas IV, Burke JF. Design of an artificial skin. I. Basic design principles. J Biomed Mater Res 1980;14(1):65–81.

24. Macadam SA, Lennox PA. Acellular dermal matrices: use in reconstructive and aesthetic breast surgery. Can J Plast Surg. Summer 2012;20(2):75–89.

25. Yannas IV, Burke JF, Gordon PL, et al. Design of an artificial skin. II. Control of chemical composition. J Biomed Mater Res 1980;14(2):107–32.

26. Dagalakis N, Flink J, Stasikelis P, et al. Design of an artificial skin. Part III. Control of pore structure. J Biomed Mater Res 1980;14(4):511–28.

27. Cheshire PA, Herson MR, Cleland H, et al. Artificial dermal templates: a comparative study of NovoSorb biodegradable Temporising matrix (BTM) and Integra((R)) dermal regeneration template (DRT). Burns 2016;42(5):1088–96.

28. Larson KW, Austin CL, Thompson SJ. Treatment of a full-thickness burn injury with novosorb biodegradable temporizing matrix and RECELL autologous skin cell suspension: a case series. J Burn Care Res 2020;41(1):215–9.

29. Malkoc A, Wong DT. Lessons learned from two survivors of greater than 90% TBSA full-thickness burn injuries using novosorb biodegradable temporizing matrix and autologous skin cell suspension, recell: a case series. J Burn Care Res 2021;42(3):577–85.

30. Alawi SA, Taqatqeh F, Matschke J, et al. Use of a collagen-elastin matrix with split-thickness skin graft for defect coverage in complex wounds. J Wound Care 2024;33(1):14–21.

31. MacEwan M, Jeng L, Kovacs T, et al. Clinical application of bioresorbable, synthetic, electrospun matrix in wound healing. Bioengineering (Basel) 2022;10(1). https://doi.org/10.3390/bioengineering10010009.

32. Ege A, Tuncay I, Ercetin O. Posterior interosseous artery flap in traumatic hand injuries. Arch Orthop Trauma Surg 2003;123(7):323–6.

33. Akdag O, Yildiran G, Sutcu M, et al. Posterior interosseous flap versus reverse adipofascial radial forearm flap for soft tissue reconstruction of dorsal hand defects. Ulus Travma Acil Cerrahi Derg 2018;24(1):43–8.

34. Sabapathy SR, Bajantri B. Indications, selection, and use of distant pedicled flap for upper limb reconstruction. Hand Clin 2014;30(2):185–99, vi.

35. Chaware SM, Dhopte AA. The superficial inferior epigastric artery based abdominal flap for reconstruction of extensive defects of the hand and forearm: a modified design with primary closure of the donor site. Ann Plast Surg 2021;86(2):162–70.

36. Gousheh J, Arasteh E, Mafi P. Super-thin abdominal skin pedicle flap for the reconstruction of hypertrophic and contracted dorsal hand burn scars. Burns 2008;34(3):400–5.

37. Urushidate S, Yotsuyanagi T, Yamauchi M, et al. Modified thin abdominal wall flap (glove flap) for the treatment of acute burns to the hands and fingers. J Plast Reconstr Aesthetic Surg 2010;63(4):693–9.

38. Ulrich D, Fuchs P, Bozkurt A, et al. Free serratus anterior fascia flap for reconstruction of hand and finger defects. Arch Orthop Trauma Surg 2010;130(2):217–22.

39. Gunasagaran J, Sian KS, Ahmad TS. Nail bed and flap reconstructions for acute fingertip injuries - a case review and report of a chemical burn injury. J Orthop Surg May-Aug 2019;27(2). 2309499019839278.

40. Agarwal P, Kumar A, Sharma D. Feasibility of type III venous flap in coverage of hand defects following trauma and burns. J Clin Orthop Trauma Oct-Dec 2016;7(Suppl 2):150–3.

41. Wolff KD, Telzrow T, Rudolph KH, et al. Isotope perfusion and infrared thermography of arterialised, venous flow-through and pedicled venous flaps. Br J Plast Surg 1995;48(2):61–70.

42. Branski LK, Mittermayr R, Herndon DN, et al. Fibrin sealant improves graft adherence in a porcine full-thickness burn wound model. Burns 2011;37(8):1360–6.

43. Schwarze H, Kuntscher M, Uhlig C, et al. Suprathel, a new skin substitute, in the management of partial-thickness burn wounds: results of a clinical study. Ann Plast Surg 2008;60(2):181–5.

44. Galati V, Vonthein R, Stang F, et al. Split thickness skin graft versus application of the temporary skin substitute suprathel in the treatment of deep dermal hand burns: a retrospective cohort study of scar elasticity and perfusion. Int J Burns Trauma 2021;11(4):312–20.

45. Wang F, Liu S, Qiu L, et al. Superthin abdominal wall glove-like flap combined with vacuum-assisted closure therapy for soft tissue reconstruction in severely burned hands or with infection. Ann Plast Surg 2015;75(6):603–6.

46. Harrison DH, Parkhouse N. Experience with upper extremity burns. the mount vernon experience. Hand Clin 1990;6(2):191–209.

47. Sungur N, Ulusoy MG, Boyacgil S, et al. Kirschner-wire fixation for postburn flexion contracture deformity and consequences on articular surface. Ann Plast Surg 2006;56(2):128–32.

48. Burm JS, Chung CH, Oh SJ. Fist position for skin grafting on the dorsal hand: I. Analysis of length of the dorsal hand surgery in hand positions. Plast Reconstr Surg 1999;104(5):1350–5.

49. Gravante G, Di Fede MC, Araco A, et al. A randomized trial comparing ReCell system of

epidermal cells delivery versus classic skin grafts for the treatment of deep partial thickness burns. Burns 2007;33(8):966–72.

50. Braza ME, Fahrenkopf MP. Split-thickness skin grafts. StatPearls 2023.

51. Nappi JF, Falcone RE, Ruberg RL. Meshed skin grafts versus sheet skin grafts on a contaminated bed. J Dermatol Surg Oncol 1984;10(5):380–1.

52. Yuste V, Delgado J, Agullo A, et al. Development of an integrative algorithm for the treatment of various stages of full-thickness burns of the first commissure of the hand. Burns 2017;43(4):812–8.

53. Baker PA, Watson SB. Functional gracilis flap in thenar reconstruction. J Plast Reconstr Aesthetic Surg 2007;60(7):828–34.

54. Pan CH, Chuang SS, Yang JY. Thirty-eight free fasciocutaneous flap transfers in acute burned-hand injuries. Burns 2007;33(2):230–5.

55. Coskunfirat OK, Ozkan O. Reversed anterior interosseous flap. J Plast Reconstr Aesthetic Surg 2006;59(12):1336–41.

56. Lu LJ, Gong X, Liu ZG, et al. Antebrachial reverse island flap with pedicle of posterior interosseous artery: a report of 90 cases. Br J Plast Surg 2004; 57(7):645–52.

57. Banis JC. Glabrous skin grafts for plantar defects. Foot Ankle Clin 2001;6(4):827–37, viii.

58. Germann GK, Reichenberger M. The burned hand. In: Scott W, Wolfe WCP, Kozin SH, et al, editors. Green's operative hand surgery. 8th edition. Phliadelphia, PA: Elsevier; 2022. p. 2121–52.

59. Greyson MA, Wilkens SC, Sood RF, et al. Five essential principles for first web space reconstruction in the burned hand. Plast Reconstr Surg 2020;146(5): 578e–87e.

60. Yang C, Yang Y, Zhong W, et al. Comparison study of 5-flap Z-plasty and double Z-plasty for interdigital pocket web contractures. J Hand Surg Am 2023. https://doi.org/10.1016/j.jhsa.2022.11.011.

61. Brown M, Chung KC. Postburn contractures of the hand. Hand Clin 2017;33(2):317–31. https://doi.org/10.1016/j.hcl.2016.12.005.

62. Barret JP, Desai MH, Herndon DN. The isolated burned palm in children: epidemiology and long-term sequelae. Plast Reconstr Surg 2000;105(3): 949–52.

63. Kurtzman LC, Stern PJ. Upper extremity burn contractures. Hand Clin 1990;6(2):261–79.

64. Sheridan RL, Hurley J, Smith MA, et al. The acutely burned hand: management and outcome based on a ten-year experience with 1047 acute hand burns. J Trauma 1995;38(3):406–11.

65. Mick JE, Reswick JB, Hager DL. The mechanism of the intrinsic-minus finger: a biomechanical study. J Hand Surg Am 1978;3(4):333–41.

66. Adani R, Marcoccio I, Tarallo L. Flap coverage of dorsum of hand associated with extensor tendons injuries: a completely vascularized single-stage reconstruction. Microsurgery 2003;23(1):32–9.

67. Davami B, Pourkhameneh G. Correction of severe postburn claw hand. Tech Hand Up Extrem Surg 2011;15(4):260–4.

68. Skoff H, Skoff H. The psychological and somatic consequences of digital amputation. Plast Reconstr Surg Glob Open 2022;10(6):e4387.

69. Graham D, Bhardwaj P, Sabapathy SR. Secondary thumb reconstruction in a mutilated hand. Hand Clin 2016;32(4):533–47.

70. Mehrabi A, Falakdami A, Mollaei A, et al. A systematic review of self-esteem and related factors among burns patients. Ann Med Surg (Lond) 2022;84:104811.

71. Issler-Fisher AC, Waibel JS, Donelan MB. Laser modulation of hypertrophic scars: technique and practice. Clin Plast Surg 2017;44(4):757–66.

Health Policy Implications of Digital Replantation

Zhixue Lim, MBChB, BMedSc, MRCS[a],
Sandeep Jacob Sebastin, MMed (Surgery), MCh (Plastic Surgery)[a],*, Kevin C. Chung, MD, MS[b]

KEYWORDS

• Digit • Finger • Hand • Amputation • Replantation • Surgeon motivation

KEY POINTS

• Patients rarely present with an ideal amputation that matches textbook indications for replantation.
• The success of replantation is strongly linked to surgeon proficiency and volume, and simply centralizing services does not seem effective to resolve this fundamental issue.
• Surgeon willingness and learned expertise is the main determinant in the choice between revision amputation and replantation; amputation seems to be favored in view of relatively low financial incentives associated with replantation procedures.

BACKGROUND

Hand injuries are extremely common and pose a worldwide burden. In the United States, nearly 45,000 digital amputations are recorded each year.[1–3] These devastating injuries predominantly affect the younger working population, resulting in significant morbidity and it is imperative to ensure that these patients receive optimal care. The 2 main options for managing these injuries are revision amputations or replantations, and although there is an exhaustive list of indications or contraindications to aid the surgeon in selecting the right procedure for the right patient, the decision-making process is complex. The course of action for certain scenarios such as multiple finger, thumb, or pediatric amputations are clear. However, there are reservations about replanting single-digit distal amputations or amputations proximal to the flexor digitorum superficialis (FDS) tendon insertion.[4,5] In addition, considerations related to both the surgeon and patient may play a pivotal role in the decision-making process. Though the factors mentioned earlier have remained consistent, the perplexing decline in digit replantation attempts has become increasingly evident over the past 2 decades, giving rise to significant concerns.[6] Despite the advocacy for centralization and regionalization endeavors in the context of hand trauma, the fundamental landscape and lackluster attitudes toward digital amputations remain unchanged.[7] In this article, we aim to unravel the complexities and examine factors regarding the dwindling digital replantation numbers.

IS REPLANTATION BETTER THAN REVISION AMPUTATION?

Yes. Although there is ample evidence to support the favorable outcomes of digital replantations compared to revision amputations, skepticism persists within the hand surgery community. To convince hand surgeons to undertake this challenging procedure, we must clearly demonstrate the distinct advantages of replantation over revision amputation. The reported survival rates of digits following digit replantation range from 57% to 92%.[5,8–10] However, relying solely on the viability of digits as the measure of replantation

[a] Department of Hand & Reconstructive Microsurgery, National University Hospital, Level 11, National University Health System Tower Block, 1E Kent Ridge Road, 119228, Singapore; [b] Section of Plastic Surgery, Department of Surgery, University of Michigan Hospital, 1500 E Medical Center Drive, 2130 Taubman Center, Ann Arbor, MI 48109, USA
* Corresponding author.
E-mail address: sandeepsebastin@gmail.com

Clin Plastic Surg 51 (2024) 553–558
https://doi.org/10.1016/j.cps.2024.02.017
0094-1298/24/© 2024 Elsevier Inc. All rights reserved.

success is overly simplistic. Traditionally, distal digital replantation has been infrequently performed due to the perception that the functional impact of a missing fingertip is negligible. Moreover, it was also because of assertions that avoiding certain replantations is justified by pointing to the potential economic and social burden on patients; this concept is not substantiated by data.[11,12] The mantra of not replanting amputations proximal to the FDS insertion, advocated in the past, was not supported by comparative data and should be revisited.[13,14]

The clinical outcomes of replantation against revision amputations have been thoroughly evaluated, and it demonstrates that replantation fares significantly better in both functional and patient-reported outcomes (PROs).[15] This remains valid even in the context of distal replantation involving a single digit. A systematic review of 2273 distal replantations revealed a high success rate of 86% done by expert surgeons and reported relatively uncommon complications of pulp atrophy and nail deformity.[9] Furthermore, a recent meta-analysis comparing digital replantation to revision amputation demonstrated that even single non-thumb digital amputations yielded superior scores on the Disability of Arm, Shoulder and Hand Questionnaire and the Michigan Hand Questionnaire.[10]

It is important to acknowledge that inappropriate surgery can put a patient at unnecessary risk and may not be cost effective. However, in the case of young and physically active workers, favorable outcomes can be achieved through replantation procedures. The restoration of appearance and function of a successfully replanted digit has superior patient satisfaction and confers long-term improvement to quality of life.[16] In terms of cost, digital replantation has also been shown to be cost effective compared to revision amputation in motivated patients.[16]

Despite robust evidence demonstrating superiority of replantation over revision amputation in both functional and PROs, there persists a disparity between the number of traumatic digit amputations and the rate of replantation attempts.

ARE DIGITAL REPLANTATION'S TECHNICALLY CHALLENGING?

Indeed, these procedures pose technical challenges that a microsurgical model cannot fully replicate. The first challenge arises in the emergency department during the determination of zone of injury, which is often underestimated. Second, the procedure's complexity is further compounded by the fractures, concomitant flexor and extensor tendon injuries, and ischemia of the digit. Third, the task of locating suitable veins for sufficient drainage adds to the overall procedural difficulty. Lastly, exacerbating the situation, most of these surgeries are performed in the middle of the night when fatigue may play a role.

HOW CAN THE SURGERY BE MADE EASIER?

Numerous tips and tricks on steps of replantation surgeries have been published and are widely available.[17–19] Unfortunately, no amount of microsurgical simulation training or reading can fully prepare an individual for replantation surgery. To alleviate the challenges of performing digital replantations, it becomes evident that only real-world practice and the application of Anders Ericsson's concept of 10,000 hours of deliberate practice can enable a smooth ascent up the learning curve.[20] As the saying goes, familiarity breeds success, and it is well established that a surgeon's proficiency is strongly correlated with positive replantation outcomes.[21]

IS THERE EVIDENCE TO SUGGEST HIGH VOLUMES INCREASE SUCCESS RATE IN REPLANTATION?

Yes, the relationship between procedure volume and positive outcomes for replantation is evident in existing literature. High-volume surgeons and centers consistently achieve greater success rates, particularly in more complex surgeries like replantation.[22,23] Asian centers, in particular, are known for their higher volumes of replantation surgery. For instance, in a systematic review of digital replantations, Sebastin and Chung reported an impressive 86% success rate in 2273 distal replantation's, with a significant proportion (70%) of these procedures performed in Asia.[9] Similarly, Stone and colleagues reported an 85.3% success rate in a sample of 717 patients, with 87.9% of these procedures occurring in Asia.[10] In contrast, Fufa and colleagues[8] evaluated a series of 135 digit replantations from 2 academic level I trauma hospital in the United States. and found a lower success rate of only 57%. The higher microsurgical success rates of the Asian centers are likely attributed to the greater volume of procedures they perform, which has also contributed to Asia's leadership in numerous microsurgical advancements over the last 2 decades.

Furthermore, the direct correlation between surgical volume and operative proficiency has also been evaluated. In a study that assessed surgeons' operative proficiency in digital replantation and revascularization procedures, it was observed that the operative proficiency scores among attending surgeons in a tertiary academic center varied substantially, and greater proficiency was linked to improved outcomes.[21] Consequently, if we continue to avoid these procedures, there is a risk that both the competence of surgeons and the standard of care can deteriorate, potentially leading to situations where even the most favorable amputation injuries may not be managed successfully. Therefore, we advocate that all borderline cases should be given an opportunity to be replanted and carefully examined under the microscope before a definitive decision is made. This will accelerate the process for the development of a competent microsurgeon as well as offer the patients a fair chance of having their digits replanted.

WHAT ARE THE CURRENT TRENDS IN REPLANTATION AND THE REASONS BEHIND DWINDLING NUMBERS?

In the United States, the number of hospitals performing replantation procedures has been steadily declining, with most hospitals conducting fewer than 10 procedures per year.[24] In addition, only a minority of hand surgeons perform finger replantation at 15% of American hospitals. To be fair, this decline coincides with a decrease in the incidence of non-fatal work-related injuries, likely attributed to the improvement in safety regulations and rapid technological advancements that have transformed job landscapes in many developed nations.[25] However, alongside these external factors, there has been a shift in attitudes among surgeons; the decline in rates of digital replantation has outpaced the reduction in the number of injuries. In an anonymous survey conducted among members of the American Society for Surgery of the Hand members, only 56% of respondents indicated that they performed replantation, with a majority performing less than 5 per year.[26] A similar downward trend of decline is observed in other developed Western countries, including Canada and Germany.[27,28] The underlying reasons for these trends are likely complex and multifactorial.

With the introduction of super-microsurgery by Koshima and colleagues,[29] which entails anastomoses as small as 0.3 mm, there exists a logical inclination to expand the boundaries of complex replantation procedures. However, the prevailing trend appears in the opposite direction. The dwindling attempts lead us to posit that the reluctance of surgeons may be the pivotal factor. If allowed to perpetuate, this situation will undoubtedly hinder a surgeon's ability to amass an adequate caseload for achieving proficiency. Some authors have voiced concerns in line with this sentiment, warning that the declining number of digital replantation in the United States. could result in reduced confidence and experience in microsurgery among practicing hand surgeons and those in training.[18,26]

We believe that the primary factor contributing to the reduced volume of replantation procedures is the willingness (or reluctance) of surgeons. A recent study on hand surgeon's dissatisfaction has revealed that call schedules and financial incentives for on-call duties play a role. The top concerns of hand surgeons taking on-call responsibilities include insufficient compensation, burnout, and high call frequency.[30] Another survey indicated that 90% of hand surgeons would be more willing to take calls if they received adequate call reimbursement.[7] In addition, Cho and colleagues[6] found that patients with private insurance were nearly twice as likely to undergo replantation compared to those with Medicare. This underscores the significant association between a patient's socioeconomic status and, indirectly, surgeons' reimbursement, which can influence surgical decisions and the care provided. This underscores the influence of incentives on behavior, suggesting that a revision to the compensation structure may help reverse the trend of declining replantation procedures.

Furthermore, in cases of amputation injuries where it is relatively easy to identify contraindications that might justify a decision for revision amputation, several additional factors come into play. These factors include a lack of microsurgical expertise, low financial incentives for replantation, and maldistribution of resources and systemic factors, all of which can significantly influence the ultimate surgical decision.[31–33]

In some cases, the temptation to pick revision amputation is high as it allows rapid return to work. In others, cultural beliefs may motivate the patient and surgeon to opt for replantation. For instance, Confucianism views the body as a sacred gift owned by one's parents and they must be intact at death.[34] Additionally, in Japanese culture, practices like 'Yubitsume,' ritualistic self-amputation often associated with the Yakuza (Japanese mafia), may influence Japanese patients' choices.[35] Historically, to avoid association with the clan, patients from those regions may be more motivated to have their digits replanted. However, these views are largely obsolete and less relevant in contemporary times. The main reasons for the greater replantation attempts in Asia are likely attributed to the strong culture established by the pioneering microsurgeons in Asia such as Tamai and Onji.[36] These centers are still helmed by second-generation leaders who uphold the same belief, which reinforces the strong impetus for replantation.

Stigmatization is another commonly cited reason for opting for replantation over revision amputation. Recently, Bettlach and colleagues[37] studied stigmatization related to digital amputations and while it concluded that it is a not highly stigmatizing condition, careful evaluation of the data showed that younger age, lower education, and workers' compensation cases were associated with significantly worse stigmatizing experiences after digital amputation. These findings suggest that patients with these characteristics may benefit from replantation procedures.

CENTRALIZATION: A VIABLE OPTION?

The proposition of centralization, which concentrates amputation cases under the care of specialized and motivated surgeons, was touted as a mean to increase replantation rates and improve patients' outcomes. This notion finds substantial support in the findings of a study by Hustedt and colleagues,[23] which demonstrated that amputation injuries presented to a high-volume centers and treated by high-volume surgeons were 2.5 times more likely to achieve a successful replantation. Richards and colleagues[38] also pointed out that the increasing trend of finger amputation injuries, which stands in contrast to a decline in replantation surgeries, underscores the necessity for centralization to better meet patients' needs.

However, despite centralization efforts and widespread availability of microvascular services at level 1 trauma centers throughout United States, data reveal a decrease in rate of replantation across all hospital types.[6] This trend deviates from the anticipated increase in volume that centralization should bring about, suggesting that the main underlying reason may be rooted in human factors such as a surgeon's willingness.

WHAT ARE SOME POSSIBLE SOLUTIONS TO ENCOURAGE REPLANTATION?

As previously discussed, we have emphasized the need for a revision to the compensation structure, which could help reverse the declining trend of replantation procedures. Furthermore, it is essential that the health care system should adapt to offer greater support to hand surgeons engaged in replantation surgeries. This includes facilitating flexible work arrangements and ensuring fair reimbursement that acknowledges and rewards their dedication and hard work. Another crucial point to address is the surgeon's attitude and reluctance. We believe that this may be rectified with

a cultural shift within the microsurgical department, like what has been championed by Tamai and Onji. Effective leadership within a department fosters a culture whereby replantation is not regarded as a thankless task but as a procedure performed with a sincere commitment to improve patients' outcomes. Shauver[39] and Chung and colleagues demonstrated the link between varying attitude and decision to replant between Japanese and American hand surgeons when surgeons were asked if they would attempt replantation based on various clinical pictures.

The current efforts to boost replantation rates should focus on training of surgical residents and fellows. It is crucial to inspire young surgeons to embrace the challenges of complex microsurgical reconstructive procedures and provide them opportunities to witness their own long-term results. The learning curve for acquiring necessary skills to perform successful replantation is typically during residency and fellowship years. We believe that a specialist with inadequate exposure to replantation cases will always tend to shy away from such procedures.

SUMMARY

We need to move away from the obfuscation of unfavorable anatomy and bad injury factors such as contraindications to replant and avoid prevarication when counseling patients on the expected course of rehabilitation and outcome of a replant. Patients rarely present with an ideal amputation that matches textbook indications for replantation and most challenges can be overcome with good surgical technique. Such expertise is achievable only through the skills of a well-trained microsurgeon. Therefore, we should not avoid demanding replantation cases and should instead embrace them as opportunities to learn from experience. At the health system level, greater efforts should be made to acknowledge and appreciate the work of surgeons who undertake these challenging procedures.

CLINICS CARE POINTS

- There is ample evidence to support favorable outcomes of digital replantations over revision amputations including functional and patient-reported outcomes.

- Despite robust evidence demonstrating superiority of replantation over revision amputations, the main underlying reason behind the disparity of traumatic digit amputations and the rate of replantation attempts is rooted in human factors such as surgeon's willingness.

- Revision to the compensation structure for surgeons can help reverse the declining trend of replantation procedures.

- The key to reverse the trend remains inspiring young surgeons and focusing of training of surgical residents and fellows to embrace the challenges of complex microsurgical reconstructive procedures.

DISCLOSURE

The authors of this article declare that they have no financial interests or conflicts that could influence the views or conclusions presented in this article. No external funding or financial support was received for this study. The authors have no affiliations with organizations or entities that may have a direct or indirect interest in the subject matter discussed in this article. This work has not been previously published or submitted for publication elsewhere.

REFERENCES

1. Renfro KN, Eckhoff MD, Trevizo GAG, et al. Traumatic finger amputations: epidemiology and mechanism of injury, 2010-2019. HAND 2022. 155894472211228.

2. Reid DBC, Shah KN, Eltorai AEM, et al. Epidemiology of finger amputations in the united states from 1997 to 2016. J Hand Surg Glob Online 2019;1(2):45–51.

3. Conn JM, Annest JL, Ryan GW, et al. Non–work-related finger amputations in the United States, 2001-2002. Ann Emerg Med 2005;45(6):630–5.

4. Urbaniak JR, Roth JH, Nunley JA, et al. The results of replantation after amputation of a single finger. J Bone Joint Surg Am 1985;67(4):611–9.

5. Waikakul S, Sakkarnkosol S, Vanadurongwan V, et al. Results of 1018 digital replantations in 552 patients. Injury 2000;31(1):33–40.

6. Cho HE, Zhong L, Kotsis SV, et al. Finger replantation optimization study (FRONT): update on national trends. J Hand Surg 2018;43(10):903–12.e1.

7. Eberlin KR, Payne DES, McCollam SM, et al. Hand trauma network in the United States: assh member perspective over the last decade. J Hand Surg 2021;46(8):645–52.

8. Fufa D, Calfee R, Wall L, et al. Digit replantation: experience of two u.s. academic level-i trauma centers. J Bone Jt Surg 2013;95(23):2127–34.

9. Sebastin SJ, Chung KC. A Systematic review of the outcomes of replantation of distal digital amputation. Plast Reconstr Surg 2011;128(3):723–37.

10. Stone N, Shah A, Chin B, et al. Comparing digital replantation versus revision amputation patient reported outcomes for traumatic digital amputations of the hand: a systematic review and meta-analysis. Microsurgery 2021;41(5):488–97.

11. Morrison WA, O'Brien BM, MacLeod AM. Evaluation of digital replantation–a review of 100 cases. Orthop Clin North Am 1977;8(2):295–308.

12. Weiland AJ, Villarreal-Rios A, Kleinert HE, et al. Replantation of digits and hands: analysis of surgical techniques and functional results in 71 patients with 86 replantations. Clin Orthop 1978;133:195–204.

13. Tamai S. Twenty years' experience of limb replantation—review of 293 upper extremity replants. J Hand Surg 1982;7(6):549–56.

14. Urbaniak JR. To replant or not to replant? That is not the question. J Hand Surg 1983;8(5):507–8.

15. Chung KC, Yoon AP, Malay S, et al. Patient-reported and functional outcomes after revision amputation and replantation of digit amputations: the FRANCHISE multicenter international retrospective cohort study. JAMA Surg 2019;154(7):637.

16. Yoon AP, Mahajani T, Hutton DW, et al, For the Finger Replantation and Amputation Challenges in Assessing Impairment, Satisfaction, and Effectiveness (FRANCHISE) Group. Cost-effectiveness of finger replantation compared with revision amputation. JAMA Netw Open 2019;2(12):e1916509.

17. Ono S, Chung KC. Efficiency in digital and hand replantation. Clin Plast Surg 2019;46(3):359–70.

18. Sabapathy SR, Venkatramani H, Bharathi RR, et al. Replantation surgery. J Hand Surg 2011;36(6):1104–10.

19. Morrison WA, McCombe D. Digital replantation. Hand Clin 2007;23(1):1–12.

20. Ericsson KA, Krampe RT, Tesch-Römer C. The role of deliberate practice in the acquisition of expert performance. Psychol Rev 1993;100(3):363–406.

21. Yoon AP, Kane RL, Wang L, et al. Variation in surgeon proficiency scores and association with digit replantation outcomes. JAMA Netw Open 2021; 4(10):e2128765.

22. Brown M, Lu Y, Chung KC, et al. Annual hospital volume and success of digital replantation. Plast Reconstr Surg 2017;139(3):672–80.

23. Hustedt JW, Bohl DD, Champagne L. The detrimental effect of decentralization in digital replantation in the United States: 15 years of evidence from the national inpatient sample. J Hand Surg 2016;41(5):593–601.

24. Chung KC, Kowalski CP, Walters MR. Finger replantation in the United States: rates and resource use from the 1996 healthcare cost and utilization project. J Hand Surg 2000;25(6):1038–42.

25. Brown J., Nearly 50 years of occupational safety and health data: beyond the Numbers: U.S. Bureau of Labor Statistics, Available at: https://www.bls.gov/opub/btn/volume-9/nearly-50-years-of-occupational-safety-and-health-data.htm, 2020. Accessed August 12, 2023.

26. Payatakes AH, Zagoreos NP, Fedorcik GG, et al. Current practice of microsurgery by members of the american society for surgery of the hand. J Hand Surg 2007;32(4):541–7.

27. Solaja O, Retrouvey H, Baltzer H. Trends in digital replantation: 10 years of experience at a large canadian tertiary care center: les tendances de la replantation digitale : dix ans d'expérience d'un grand centre canadien de soins tertiaires. Plast Surg 2021;29(1):21–9.

28. Kükrek H, Moog P, Nedeoglo E, et al. The declining number of finger replantations in Germany. Ann Plast Surg 2022;88(1):44–8.

29. Koshima I, Yamamoto T, Narushima M, et al. Perforator flaps and supermicrosurgery. Clin Plast Surg 2010;37(4):683–9.

30. Douleh DG, Ipaktchi K, Lauder A. Hand call practices and satisfaction: survey results from hand surgeons in the United States. J Hand Surg 2022; 47(11):1120. e1-e9.

31. Mahmoudi E, Chung KC. Effect of hospital volume on success of thumb replantation. J Hand Surg 2017;42(2):96–103.e5.

32. Mahmoudi E, Swiatek PR, Chung KC, et al. Racial variation in treatment of traumatic finger/thumb amputation: a national comparative study of replantation and revision amputation. Plast Reconstr Surg 2016;137(3):576e–85e.

33. Mahmoudi E, Squitieri L, Maroukis BL, et al. Care transfers for patients with upper extremity trauma: influence of health insurance type. J Hand Surg 2016;41(4):516–25.e3. d.

34. Badanta B, González-Cano-Caballero M, Suárez-Reina P, et al. How does confucianism influence health behaviors, health outcomes and medical decisions? a scoping review. J Relig Health 2022;61(4):2679–725.

35. Bosmia A, Griessenauer CJ, Tubbs S. Yubitsume: ritualistic self-amputation of proximal digits among the yakuza. J Inj Violence Res 2014;6(2):54–6.

36. Tamai S. History of microsurgery. Plast Reconstr Surg 2009;124:e282–94.

37. Bettlach CR, Gibson E, Daines JM, et al. The stigma of digital amputation: a survey of amputees with analysis of risk factors. J Hand Surg Eur 2022; 47(5):461–8.

38. Richards WT, Barber MK, Richards WA, et al. Hand injuries in the state of Florida, are centers of excellence needed? J Trauma Inj Infect Crit Care 2010; 68(6):1480–90.

39. Shauver MJ, Nishizuka T, Hirata H, et al. Traumatic finger amputation treatment preference among hand surgeons in the United States and Japan. Plast Reconstr Surg 2016;137(4):1193–202.

From Simple to Complex
Preserving and Reconstructing the Traumatized Thumb

Jonathan T. Bacos, MD*, Sarah E. Sasor, MD

KEYWORDS

- Thumb reconstruction • Moberg flap • Index pollicization • Distraction lengthening
- Osteoplastic reconstruction • Toe transfer

KEY POINTS

- The goals of thumb reconstruction are to restore thumb length, stability, mobility, and sensibility.
- Thumb reconstruction requires a thorough preoperative assessment of the injury, functional deficit, and potential donor sites. The patient's medical, occupation, hobbies, and expectations are considered in developing a personalized treatment plan.
- Thumb deficits can be categorized by the level of tissue loss (distal, middle, or proximal third). There are many reconstructive options for each injury level.
- Rehabilitation postsurgery is crucial to regain functionality of the reconstructed thumb.

INTRODUCTION

Traumatic thumb injuries result in significant disability, affecting a patient's livelihood and ability to perform activities of daily living. The thumb is responsible for 40% to 50% of hand function[1]; thus, there is a great incentive to preserve the thumb after injury.[2] In cases of complete thumb amputation, replantation is always considered; however, in cases where replantation is not feasible or when there is partial thumb loss, reconstruction is necessary. This article reviews reconstructive principles and operative techniques for reconstructing the traumatized thumb.

PREOPERATIVE ASSESSMENT

A thorough history, physical examination, and radiographs are required in the workup of any traumatic thumb injury. The patient's occupation, hobbies, hand dominance, and any prior trauma or surgery should be noted. Inspect for lacerations, soft tissue defects, deformity, open fractures, and contamination. Evaluate for perfusion and sensation to all aspects of the thumb. Assess active and passive range of motion, joint stability, and strength.

Examine the basilar joint—even when not acutely injured, painful arthritis or instability may preclude certain types of reconstruction. Similarly, first web-space skin deficiency or contracture should be noted–; a deficient webspace will restrict thumb opposition and abduction. The remaining digits on the hand should also be evaluated, as the functionality of a thumb depends on its ability to make useful contact with the remaining digits.

The standard 3 view (posterior–anterior, oblique, and lateral) hand radiographs are mandatory. True anterior–posterior (Robert's) and lateral (Bett's) views of the trapeziometacarpal joint are also useful.

Involve the patient in the decision process when possible. Comprehensive thumb reconstruction frequently involves multiple surgeries and extensive postoperative hand therapy. The patient and surgeon must have similar goals to ensure success.[3]

Department of Plastic Surgery, Medical College of Wisconsin, 8701 W. Watertown Plank Road, Wauwatosa, WI 53226, USA
* Corresponding author.
E-mail address: jbacos@mcw.edu

Clin Plastic Surg 51 (2024) 559–573
https://doi.org/10.1016/j.cps.2024.04.001

SURGICAL ANATOMY

The vascular supply of the thumb varies from that of other fingers in that the volar and dorsal blood supply are fairly independent. The volar surface is supplied by two palmar collateral arteries arising from the princeps pollicis artery. The dorsal blood supply is supplied by ulnar dorsocollateral and radial dorsocollateral arteries.[4–7] Injury to either arterial supply may preclude certain reconstructive options.

GOALS OF RECONSTRUCTION

The primary goals of thumb reconstruction are to restore form and function; this can be achieved with adequate bone length, stability, motion, and sensibility. Esthetic considerations are secondary.

We prefer to stratify thumb reconstruction based on the level of tissue loss with the thumb ray divided in thirds, as described by Muzaffar and colleagues.[8] The remainder of this article provides a systematic approach to thumb reconstruction based on the level of tissue loss.

Distal Third

The distal third of the thumb extends from the interphalangeal joint to the fingertip. For many patients, amputation through the distal third remains functional.[8] The main goal of distal third reconstruction is soft tissue coverage with sensate and durable tissue.

Secondary Intention and Skin Grafting

When no bone is exposed, small soft tissue defects of the distal thumb heal well by secondary intention. Healing may require weeks of local wound care, but the resultant scar is stable and sensate.[9,10] When the defect is greater than 1.5 cm^2, skin grafting can be considered. Skin grafting is an acceptable option in the patient who desires a simple solution that avoids a protracted course of local wound care. The patient *must* be counseled that graft will be insensate.

Local flaps

When the distal phalanx is exposed, flap coverage is warranted. There are multiple options available depending on the anatomy of the wound and the quality of surrounding tissue.

Volar advancement flap The Moberg neurovascular advancement flap is indicated for coverage of up to 2 cm^2 defects on the volar surface of the thumb.[11] It is a bipedicled flap raised on the ulnar and radial digital arteries. Parallel mid-lateral incisions are made from the wound distally to the digital palmar crease proximally. The incisions are dorsal to the neurovascular bundles and the bundles are elevated with the flap. The volar flap is elevated directly off the flexor retinaculum and advanced distally. Advancement is limited, but the flap provides highly sensate, glabrous skin to the defect (**Fig. 1**).

The downside of this flap is the tendency for interphalangeal joint flexion deformity if the flap is insufficiently mobilized. The flap can be islandized to gain length by incising across the digital palmar crease (superficial to the neurovascular bundles), which allows greater mobility of the flap and can be closed in a V-Y manner or with skin grafting.[12]

Homodigital collateral artery flap When phalangeal bone is exposed dorsally, the reverse-flow homodigital collateral artery flap is a reasonable reconstructive option.[4,13–16] Originally described by Brunelli and Moschella, the flap is harvested off the proximal aspect of the dorsal thumb. The flap is supplied by the respective ulnar dorsocollateral or radial dorsocollateral arteries which arise from the radial artery at the level of the first metacarpal head. The skin flap is centered over its axial blood supply, and meticulous microdissection is performed from proximal to distal, ending at the level of the mid-proximal phalanx to preserve anastomosis between the palmar and dorsal vessels. The flap is reflected into the defect, and the donor site is closed primarily. The dorsocollateral branch of the superficial radial nerve can be coapted to a volar collateral nerve to create a sensate flap.[12]

Cross-finger flaps Cross-finger flaps from the dorsal index can be used for coverage of distal thumb defects of 2 to 3 cm^2. A full-thickness skin graft is used at the donor site. This is a 2 staged reconstruction that requires flap division several weeks later (**Fig. 2**). This flap can include transposition of the dorsal sensory branch of the radial nerve to restore sensation. Owing to variable sensory recovery, an additional coaptation of the dorsal sensory branch of the index radial digital nerve to the ulnar digital nerve of the thumb has been reported and has demonstrated 2 point discrimination of 5 mm on the volar pulp.[17,18]

Heterodigital island flap The heterodigital neurovascular island flap described by Littler allows for single-staged, sensate reconstruction.[19] The donor site is based on the ulnar neurovascular bundle of either the middle or ring finger. This flap requires extensive dissection of the donor finger and the palm and, because of this, is rarely used (**Fig. 3**).[20,21]

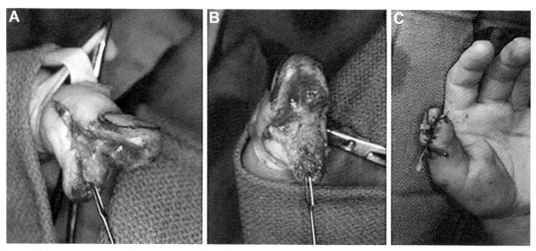

Fig. 1. Volar advancement flap used for volar oblique thumb injury. (*A, B*) Elevation of the Moberg advancement flap followed by inset over drains (*C*).

FREE TISSUE TRANSFER

Free toe pulp flaps or onycho-osteocutaneous flaps are occasionally used to reconstruct distal thumb defects. Benefits include a single-stage reconstruction with superior esthetics and functionality. This reconstruction may be considered for musicians who play string instruments and some manual laborers.[22–24] Free tissue transfer for thumb defects is more common for middle and proximal thumb defects.

Middle Third

The middle third of the thumb is located between the interphalangeal joint and the metacarpal neck. The functional outcome of thumb reconstruction at this level is affected by the bone length and thenar musculature status. Injuries proximal to the metacarpophalangeal joint result in destruction of thenar musculature and loss of opposition. Maintenance of length and opposable tripod pinch are essential in this zone.

First dorsal metacarpal artery flap

The first dorsal metacarpal artery (FDMA) or kite flap is useful to reconstruct soft tissue defects with exposed bone on the dorsal and distal aspects middle third. The flap is harvested from the dorsal surface of the index finger and is supplied by the first dorsal metacarpal artery. It can be innervated by including a branch of the superficial radial nerve.[25] Successful reconstruction with this flap requires elevating the skin flap with the underlying fascia of the first interosseous muscle incorporating the vascular pedicle. Dissection continues proximally into the anatomic snuffbox, and a subcutaneous tunnel is created between the donor site and the skin defect.[12]

A reverse-flow modification of this flap can reach the distal thumb tip. The reverse-flow flap is designed more proximal and lateral than the traditional FDMA flap and involves sectioning the ulnar and radial branches of the FDMA adjacent to their radial artery origin. This flap remains

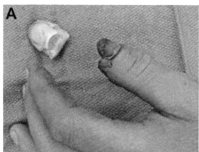
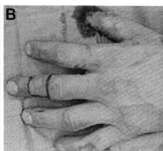
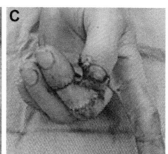

Fig. 2. Middle finger to thumb cross-finger flap for distal phalanx coverage. (*A*) The distal thumb defect and markings for flap elevation in (*B*). (*C*) Flap inset and skin grafting over the dorsal middle finger defect.

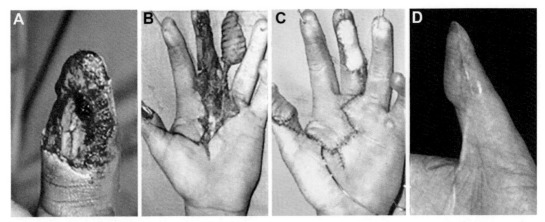

Fig. 3. Neurovascular island pedicle flap from middle finger to thumb for distal volar thumb defect. (A) The distal thumb defect followed by flap elevation in (B) and flap inset with skin grafting to the donor site defect (C). (D) The healed flap postoperatively.

perfused by deep communications between the FDMA and princeps pollicis artery (**Fig. 4**).[26]

Thumb reconstruction in the middle third is more challenging when defects include soft tissue and bone loss. Functional restoration is achieved with either an increase in the relative or absolute length of the thumb.

Webspace deepening

Increasing the *relative* length of the thumb is achieved by phalangization, where the first webspace is deepened and the thumb index interval is widened. Phalangization is most useful when

defects are limited to the distal half of the middle third. The tethering structures between the thumb and index finger rays are released and the adductor insertion is repositioned proximally onto the metacarpal shaft. This allows for better excursion and improves opposition.

Webspace deepening may also be required when first webspace contracture arises *after* thumb reconstruction. Circumvent this pitfall with edema control and protective splinting with the thumb in palmar abduction in all cases of traumatic thumb injuries.

For a contracted first webspace, there are various methods for deepening. In some cases, a linear scar

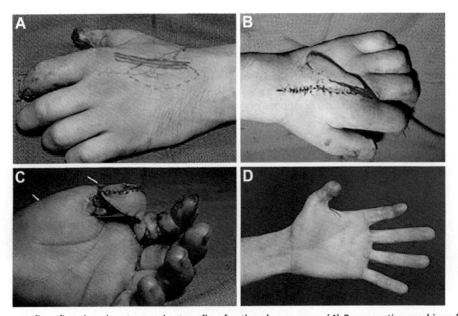

Fig. 4. Reverse-flow first dorsal metacarpal artery flap for thumb coverage. (A) Preoperative markings followed by flap elevation and donor site closure (B). Flap inset can be seen in (C) followed by delayed flap division and inset in (D).

can be improved with adjacent tissue rearrangement (Z-plasty or jumping man flaps). If there is significant scar contracture, release and resurfacing with a flap is necessary. Options include the dorsal hand rotation, reverse radial forearm, posterior interosseous, or lateral arm free flaps (**Fig. 5**).

Traumatic injuries involving the proximal aspect of the middle third of the thumb require an increase in the *absolute* length of the thumb for function. There are many options for increasing the length of the thumb including an on-top plasty from spare parts, distraction osteogenesis, and osteoplastic reconstruction.

On-top plasty

On-top plasty is a spare part surgery where the distal portion of a damaged or partially amputated finger is transferred to the remaining thumb stump. This was first described as a neurovascular pedicle transfer, but microsurgical techniques can also be utilized. Any digit may be used.[8] The amount of bone transferred should be matched to the amount of bone lost. The most critical aspect of an on-top plasty is preserving a minimum of one dorsal vein for venous outflow. A similar but distinct approach to thumb reconstruction, pollicization, entails transfer of a normally functioning digit to the thumb and involves transfer of the flexor and extensor mechanisms; these are often damaged in an on-top plasty. Pollicization will be discussed later in this article.

Distraction lengthening

Metacarpal distraction lengthening follows principles originally defined by Ilizarov[27] and was popularized for applications in thumb reconstruction by Matev.[28,29] Distraction lengthening consists of application of an external fixation device, osteotomy of the diaphysis, and then a period of bony distraction at 1 mm per day until the desired length is achieved. Metacarpal distraction requires two-thirds of the native metacarpal length but can achieve approximately 3 to 3.5 cm gain in length.[8] Although children often spontaneously ossify the

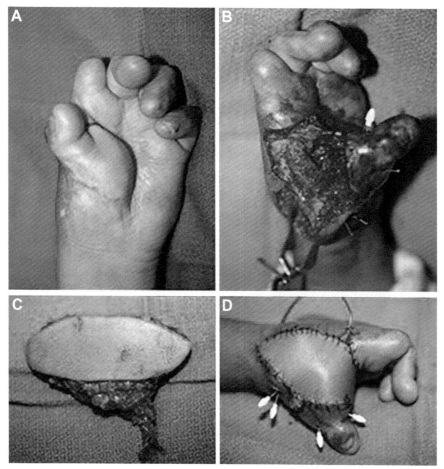

Fig. 5. Lateral arm free flap used for first webspace resurfacing following severe burn scar contracture. (A) The first webspace contracture followed by scar excision (B). Lateral arm free flap (C) inset over drains (D).

bone gap created by distraction, older patients may require bone grafting to achieve bony union.[30] For successful lengthening of the thumb, one should consider stabilizing the metacarpophalangeal joint with Kirschner wires to avoid inadvertent joint flexion with progressive lengthening.

Distraction lengthening is an imperfect solution with multiple shortcomings. The distraction process is time-consuming, requires multiple surgeries, and has a relatively high rate of pin site infection and hardware failure. Additionally, this procedure is associated with webspace creep which may require webspace deepening.[31] Furthermore, though distraction adds length to the digit, it does not address motor function, strength, or positioning. Additional surgery for tendon transfer(s) may be necessary to improve the functionality of the lengthened digit.

Osteoplastic reconstruction

Osteoplastic reconstruction is a multistage reconstruction method that combines a bone graft with a flap to lengthen the thumb remnant. Skeletal reconstruction is often achieved with iliac crest bone graft wrapped with a tubed groin flap (Fig. 6). This is followed by flap division, thinning, and pulp reconstruction with a neurovascular island flap to achieve sensibility. Many variations in osteoplastic reconstruction have been described.[32] Doi and colleagues described a single-stage procedure including iliac crest bone graft combined with a free dorsalis pedis flap.[33] One of the disadvantages of traditional osteoplastic reconstruction includes bone graft resorption. To avoid this complication, vascularized bone flaps and free toe transfers have replaced traditional osteoplastic methods of reconstruction in many centers (Fig. 7).

Sabapathy and colleagues reported a case of an individual sustaining bilateral thumb amputations just distal to the metacarpophalangeal joint (MCPJ) who underwent osteoplastic reconstruction on the right and great toe transfer on the left. Two years after the injury, there was no significant difference in the functional of the 2 thumbs; however, the patient preferred the great toe for cosmetic reasons.[34]

Toe Transfers

Wraparound toe transfer

The wraparound toe transfer was introduced by Morrison and is a hybrid of osteoplastic reconstruction and great toe transfer.[35] The operation includes the transfer of the distal half of the distal phalanx along with plantar, lateral, and dorsal tissues, including the nail. The complex is wrapped around bone graft, which spans the gap between the remaining thumb skeleton and distal phalanx

of the transferred toe. This technique is thought to decrease bone graft resorption, as it is sandwiched between two vascularized bones (Fig. 8). This flap was previously used for loss distal to the metacarpophalangeal joint but has been used for reconstruction at more proximal levels as well.[36]

Preoperative markings rely on measurements taken from the contralateral thumb to guide a narrower, more esthetic transfer. The fingernail complex can also be narrowed by resecting germinal matrix on each side. This transfer leaves medial toe skin and the distal phalanx out to the base of the toenail. The donor site may be closed by disarticulating the remaining interphalangeal joint and closing the medial skin flap primarily. Alternatively, a cross toe flap from the second toe may be used to close the donor site and preserve great toe length.[37]

Great toe transfer

The great toe-to-thumb transfer was first performed by Nicoladoni and Daumenplastik as a pedicled flap.[38] In 1969, Cobbett described microvascular toe transfers in humans[39,40] and advanced soft tissue and skeletal reconstruction of the thumb to be feasible in a single operation. The great toe transfer is technically demanding and requires familiarity with vascular anatomy of the foot.[41–44] In general, preoperative angiography of the lower extremity is not required but may be considered when the vascular status is uncertain.

The great toe flap is designed to facilitate primary closure and to avoid scars on weight-bearing areas. Typically, the incision is v-shaped, starting medially from the first webspace and extending laterally just distal to the metatarsophalangeal joint. Dissection proceeds retrograde from the first webspace to identify the arterial branches to the great and second toes and then more proximally to the dominant arterial supply. The first dorsal metatarsal artery is usually dominant and is identified by its dorsal location in relation to the intermetatarsal ligament. Greater success has been achieved using the dorsal system; however, the plantar system has been shown to be dominant in 23% of cases.[42,45] If the first plantar metatarsal artery is dominant, the dorsal dissection continues to isolate the extensor tendon and a major dorsal vein. Plantar dissection then proceeds with isolation of the flexor tendon, nerves, and plantar digital artery. Dissection of the plantar digital artery can be tedious as it may wraparound the plantar sesamoid bone of the great toe. Following isolation of nerve, tendon, artery, and vein, the metatarsophalangeal joint is disarticulated from the toe. It is preferred to preserve the volar head of the first metatarsal and sesamoid to avoid gait disturbance in toe transfer. If necessary, the dorsal

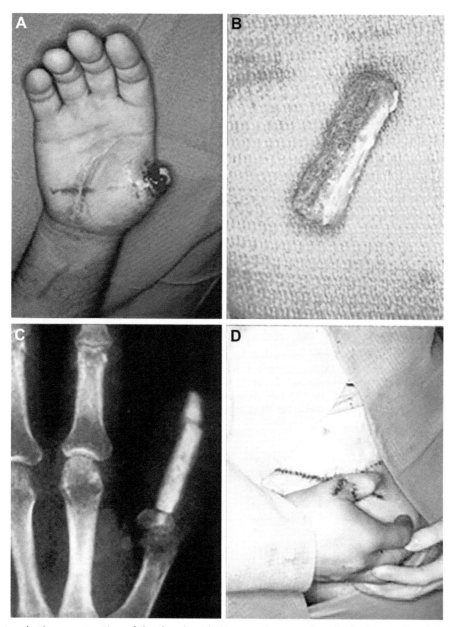

Fig. 6. Osteoplastic reconstruction of the thumb with iliac crest bone graft and tubed groin flap. (*A*) The thumb defect. Iliac crest bone graft was harvested seen in (*B*) and visualized on X-ray in (*C*). A tubed groin flap was used to provide soft tissue coverage (*D*).

75% of the metatarsal head may be removed to achieve closure of the foot.[46]

Once the great toe is harvested, it can be inset onto the thumb remnant. Multiple techniques have been described for osteosynthesis. Following bony fixation, extensor and tendon repairs are performed. The toe has an innate propensity to claw, which can be prevented with a tight extensor repair and temporary Kirschner wire fixation of the toe in extension. The dorsal radial artery is anastomosed to the great toe artery, and a large superficial vein

from the transferred toe is anastomosed to the cephalic vein. Last, the distal end of the dorsal radial nerve supplying the dorsum of the thumb is coapted to the distal branches of the deep and superficial peroneal nerve supplying the dorsum of the toe. The ulnar and radial digital nerves are repaired end to end to the corresponding nerves of the great toe.

Postoperatively, the great toe transfer requires close monitoring and will follow a postoperative protocol similar to replanted digits (**Fig. 9**).[47]

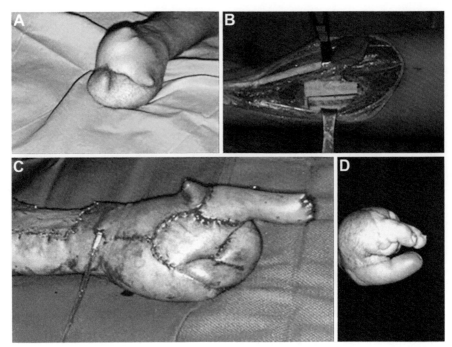

Fig. 7. Reverse radial forearm osteocutaneous flap for thumb reconstruction followed by staged second toe transfers for digit reconstruction. (*A*) A patient with traumatic amputations at the distal metacarpal level followed by groin flap coverage. He underwent reverse radial forearm osteocutaneous flap (*B*). The donor site was closed with skin grafting and the flap was closed over a drain (*C*). He subsequently underwent second-stage toe transfers to achieve pinch and grasp function (*D*).

Trimmed great toe transfer

The trimmed great toe flap is a variation of the great toe transfer that combines the functional improvements of the great toe flap with the custom site and esthetic features of the wrap-around toe technique. The great toe is 20% larger than the thumb and, with volume reduction, provides a more thumblike appearing appendage.[8] Harvesting a trimmed great toe is performed by measuring the contralateral thumb and mapping this on the toe such that size discrepancies can be marked on the medial aspect of the great toe. A reduction of both bone and soft tissue is performed including excision of medial skin and a longitudinal osteotomy to overcome size discrepancy of the new thumb.[48,49] This allows for creation of a new thumb that is as similar as possible to the contralateral thumb.[50] Of note, this method is contraindicated in children because damage to growth plates would be incurred during harvest.[51]

Second toe transfer

Second toe transfer is an alternative technique in thumb reconstruction. In contrast to the great toe, the second toe contains an extra interphalangeal joint and is smaller than the native thumb with a narrow neck, bulbous tip, and short nail. Advantages

of using the second toe for thumb reconstruction include an inconspicuous donor site deformity and minimal donor site morbidity.[52] Additionally, when patients suffer thumb amputations proximal to the metacarpal phalangeal joint, the second toe transfer may be a better option as it eliminates the donor site morbidity associated with taking the first metatarsal head.[53,54]

Drawbacks of using the second toe in thumb reconstruction include a smaller contact surface, higher rates of flexion contracture, and reduced grip and pinch strength compared to a great toe.[55] Despite these critiques, a systematic review by Lin and colleagues comparing outcomes of different toe to thumb transfers demonstrated no statistically significant difference in arc of motion, grip, and pinch strength when comparing second-to-great toe transfers.[49] Esthetic refinements of second toe- to-thumb transfer by Zhao and colleagues have a significantly improved the thumblike appearance of the second toe transfers with excellent results (**Fig. 10**).[56]

Secondary surgeries

Other procedures commonly required in patients undergoing toe transfer procedures include opponensplasty, tenolysis, arthrodesis, and pulp reduction.[57]

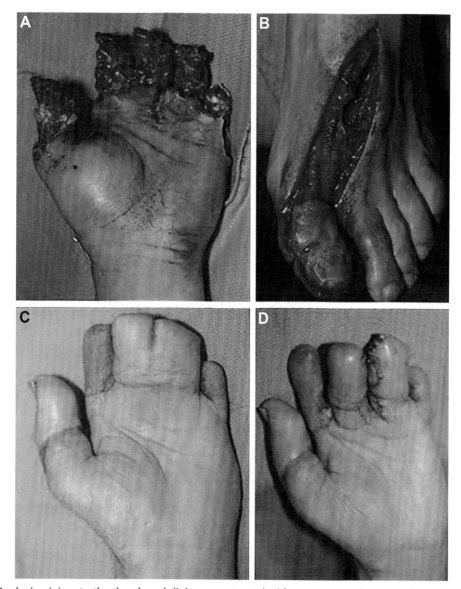

Fig. 8. Degloving injury to the thumb and digits reconstructed with a wraparound toe transfer and radial fore-arm split flap for digit coverage. (A) A crush injury and degloving of the thumb and digits. The patient underwent wraparound great toe harvest for thumb reconstruction (B) and digit coverage with a radial forearm flap (C) fol-lowed by staged radial forearm flap division and skin grafting (D).

Complications

As with all reconstructive options, toe-to-thumb transfers are not without complications. The most feared complication is vascular compromise. A systematic review including 450 toe-to-thumb transfers of many types demonstrated a mean survival rate of 96.4%.[49] This is similar to the 95% to 98% survival reported for other free flaps.[58–60] Lin and colleagues performed a multivariate analysis of 363 cases in toe-to-hand transfer and found that infection was the single greatest factor contributing to vascular compromise and re-exploration.

Higher re-exploration rates were found in acute toe transfers compared to delayed toe transfers (21.1% vs 14.9%). Delaying toe transfers until after the acute trauma improves operative outcomes.[61]

Donor site morbidity following toe transfer surgery should be discussed preoperatively. The most common donor site complications include wound dehiscence, infection, necrosis, pain, and callosity. Great toe transfers have been associated with higher morbidity than second toe transfers.[62] A few cases of painful foot neuromas have been reported which were treated with neuroma resection

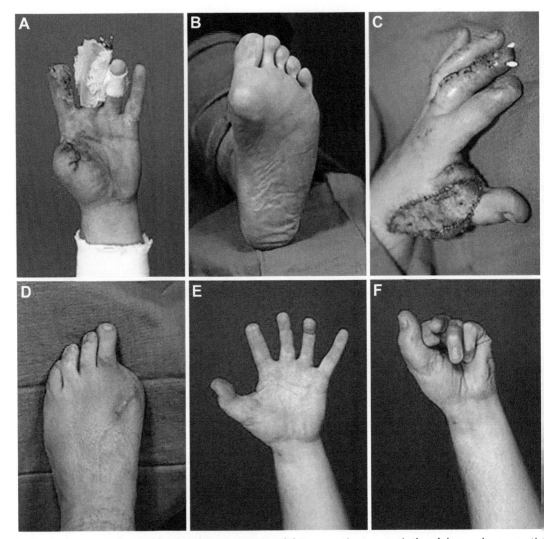

Fig. 9. Great toe transfer used for thumb reconstruction. (*A*) Preoperative traumatic thumb loss and preoperative evaluation of the left great toe donor site (*B*). Great toe transfer was performed with skin grafting (*C*). Donor site deformity can be seen in (*D*) and postoperative result in (*E*) and (*F*).

and implantation of the nerve into muscle.[63] Overall, gait tends to be minimally affected, and the donor site morbidity remains largely acceptable given the gain in hand function.

Outcomes

Overall, postoperative assessment of strength, mobility, sensibility, and hand-related quality of life is favorable in patients undergoing toe transfer operations. Patients who undergo toe transfer for thumb amputations at the metacarpophalangeal joint level report better scores in overall hand function, activities of daily living, work performance, and esthetic scores than amputation controls.[64] These outcomes are supported by a systematic review by Lin and colleagues, which demonstrated that

great toe transfer demonstrated a mean total active motion return of 58°, 84% return of grip strength, and 81% return of key pinch strength compared with those of the contralateral hand. Notably, recent report by Shaffrey and colleagues presented a patient with a 40 year follow-up after great toe-to thumb reconstruction with high esthetic and functional satisfaction validating the longevity of the reconstructive technique.[65]

Proximal Third

The proximal third of the thumb is demarcated by the level of the metacarpal neck to the carpometacarpal joint. Injury to the proximal third represents a complete loss, including loss of thenar musculature. Thumb amputations at this level typical

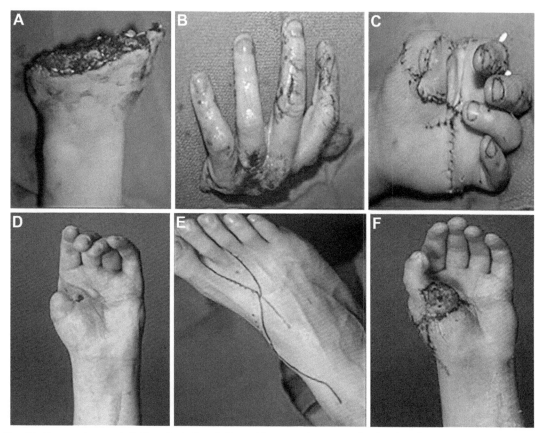

Fig. 10. Transmetacarpal digit replantation followed by second toe transfer for thumb reconstruction. (*A, B*) A transmetatarsal digit amputation. This patient underwent replantation (*C*). He had a remaining thumb defect seen in (*D*). A second toe transfer was planned with preoperative donor site markings seen in (*D*). Postoperative result seen in (*E*).

necessitate the addition of at least 5 cm of length. The primary goal of proximal thumb reconstruction is to create a stable and sensate post for pinch and opposition.[66] Options for reconstruction at this level are limited. In some scenarios, transfer of an injured digit as an on-top plasty may be performed (as was previously described); however, when this option is not available, pollicization of a normal digit should be considered.

Pollicization
Commonly used to treat congenital thumb hypoplasia, pollicization is a useful reconstructive option in setting of traumatic loss of the thumb at the level of the carpometacarpal (CMC) joint.[67,68] Pollicization transposes a nearby digit—most often the adjacent index finger—to the thumb position. The transposed digit is mobilized on its neurovascular bundle and reoriented in 45° of abduction and approximately 100° of pronation.[69] The common digital nerve must be separated intraneurally. The ulnar digital artery can be divided if the radial digital artery perfuses the digit.

Alternatively, the radial digital artery to the adjacent middle finger can be divided and the common digital artery to the second webspace can be transferred with the index finger. Transfer of the index finger allows for webspace deepening via excision of excess metacarpal and is considered an esthetic reconstruction (**Fig. 11**).[70] Technical details of the surgery are well described in many studies.[71,72]

Possible complications of pollicization include kinking, twisting or compression of the pedicle, delayed union or nonunion, and the occasional need for tenolysis or opponensplasty. For proximal amputations (distal to the carpometacarpal joint with intact intrinsic thumb muscles) toe-to-thumb transfer may still be performed. Both pollicization and toe-to-hand transfer have satisfactory motor and sensory outcomes.[73,74]

Prosthetics
Prosthetic devices play a limited role in thumb reconstruction. In general, prosthetic devices are esthetic in nature and have minimal function.

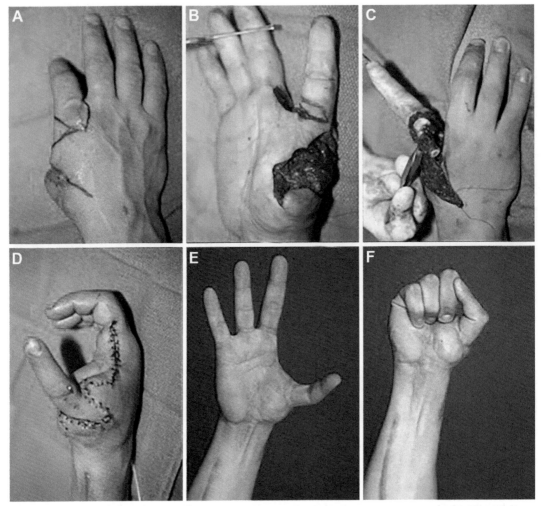

Fig. 11. Index pollicization following traumatic thumb injury. (*A*) Donor site markings for index finger pollicization. (*B*) The flap elevation followed by index finger transfer in (*C*). The digit is inset in palmar abduction and pronation (*D*). Postoperative index pollicization (*E*) with key pinch demonstrated in (*F*).

Nonetheless, restoring normal appearance can improve body image and psychological well-being after trauma.[75]

Previously, at least 1 cm of proximal phalanx was required for prosthetic fitting. Prosthetics for total thumb loss required a glove to be worn over the palm.[8]

Recent advances in bone-anchored devices provide an alternative to conventional socket prostheses. Bone-anchored devices allow for firm attachment of the prosthetic to the body with freer movement. Li and colleagues report a series of 13 patients treated with osteointegrated thumb prosthesis and found that active users achieved 66% of grip strength and 71% of lateral pinch strength compared with the unaffected side, which is comparable to great toe-to-thumb transfer.[76] Additionally, osteointegrated prostheses translate vibration

and pressure via osseoperception. However, there is currently limited adoption of this bone-anchored thumb prosthesis, which may in part be due to concerns regarding mechanical failure, the need for ongoing maintenance and the risk of infection.

SUMMARY

Traumatic injuries to the thumb can dramatically alter one's ability to complete basic tasks that rely on grip, grasp, and coordination. Reconstruction of function directly impacts a patient's independence, quality of life, and ability to partake in work, hobbies, and activities of daily living. The goal of thumb reconstruction is to preserve function, sensibility, stability, and strength. Surgeons must identify traumatized structures and develop a comprehensive plan tailored to the injury and the patient.

CLINICS CARE POINTS

- Thumb replantation should always be considered for complete, traumatic amputations. When patient or injury factors prohibit replantation, thumb reconstruction is necessary. The goals of reconstruction are to maintain bone length, stability, motion, and sensibility.

- Successful thumb reconstruction requires a thorough preoperative assessment of the defect, surrounding tissues, and the availability of suitable donor tissue. The patient's occupation, hobbies, and medical history are considered to formulate a personalized treatment plan.

- Thumb reconstruction is technically demanding, and multiple operations are often required. Careful patient selection is essential and thorough preoperative counseling is essential.

ACKNOWLEDGMENTS

The authors thank Dr James Sanger, Hani Matloub, and John Yousif for the clinical photographs included in this article.

DISCLOSURE

The authors have nothing to disclose.

REFERENCES

1. Bunnell S. Reconstruction of the thumb. Am J Surg 1958;95(2):168–72.
2. Littler JW. On making a thumb: one hundred years of surgical effort. J Hand Surg Am 1976;1(1):35–51.
3. Eaton CJ. Thumb reconstruction. In: Thorne CH, Beasley RW, Aston SJ, et al, editors. Grabb and smith's plastic surgery. Philadelphia: Lippincott Williams & Wilkins; 2006.
4. Brunelli F, Vigasio A, Valenti P, et al. Arterial anatomy and clinical application of the dorsoulnar flap of the thumb. J Hand Surg Am 1999;24(4):803–11.
5. Ames EL, Bissonnette M, Acland R, et al. Arterial anatomy of the thumb. J Hand Surg Br 1993;18(4):427–36.
6. Miletin J, Sukop A, Baca V, et al. Arterial supply of the thumb: systemic review. Clin Anat 2017;30(7):963–73.
7. Matloub HS, Strathy KM, Sanger JR, et al. Venous anatomy of the thumb. J Hand Surg Am 1991;16(6):1063–9.
8. Muzaffar AR, Chao JJ, Friedrich JB, et al. Posttraumatic thumb reconstruction. Plast Reconstr Surg 2005;116(5):103e–22e.
9. Bickel KD, Dosanjh A. Fingertip reconstruction. J Hand Surg Am 2008;33(8):1417–9.
10. Vedder BN, Friedrich JB. Plastic surgery. Hand and Upper Limb 2017;6. Elsevier.
11. Heitmann C, Levin LS. Alternatives to thumb replantation. Plast Reconstr Surg 2002;110(6):1492–503. quiz 1504-5.
12. Rehim SA, Chung KC. Local flaps of the hand. Hand Clin 2014;30(2):137–51.
13. Brunelli F. Le lambeau dorso-cubital du pouce [Dorso-ulnar thumb flap]. Ann Chir Main Memb Super 1993;12(2):105–14.
14. Moschella F, Cordova A, Pirrelo R, et al. Anatomic basis for the dorsal radial flap of the thumb: clinical applications. Surg Radiol Anat 1996;18(3):179–81.
15. Moschella F, Cordova A. Reverse homodigital dorsal radial flap of the thumb. Plast Reconstr Surg 2006;117(3):920–6.
16. Terán P, Carnero S, Miranda R, et al. Refinements in dorsoulnar flap of the thumb: 15 cases. J Hand Surg Am 2010;35(8):1356–9.
17. Hastings H. 2nd, Dual innervated index to thumb cross finger or island flap reconstruction. Microsurgery 1987;8(3):168–72.
18. Lim JX, Chung KC. VY advancement, thenar flap, and cross-finger flaps. Hand Clin 2020;36(1):19–32.
19. Littler JW. The neurovascular pedicle method of digital transposition for reconstruction of the thumb. Plast Reconstr Surg (1946) 1953;12(5):303–19.
20. Adani R, Squarzina PB, Castagnetti C, et al. A comparative study of the heterodigital neurovascular island flap in thumb reconstruction, with and without nerve reconnection. J Hand Surg Br 1994;19(5):552–9.
21. Xarchas KC, Tilkeridis KE, Pelekas SI, et al. Littler's flap revisited: an anatomic study, literature review, and clinical experience in the reconstruction of large thumb-pulp defects. Med Sci Monit 2008;14(11):CR568–73.
22. Yan H, Ouyang Y, Chi Z, et al. Digital pulp reconstruction with free neurovascular toe flaps. Aesthetic Plast Surg 2012;36(5):1186–93.
23. Foucher G, Nagel D, Briand E. Microvascular great toenail transfer after conventional thumb reconstruction. Plast Reconstr Surg 1999;103(2):570–6.
24. Del Pinal F, Moraleda E, de Piero GH, et al. Onycho-osteo-cutaneous defects of the thumb reconstructed by partial hallux transfer. J Hand Surg Am 2014;39(1):29–36.
25. Foucher G, Braun JB. A new island flap transfer from the dorsum of the index to the thumb. Plast Reconstr Surg 1979;63(3):344–9.
26. Checcucci G, Galeano M, Zucchini M, et al. Reverse flow first dorsal metacarpal artery flap for covering

the defect of distal thumb. Microsurgery 2014;34(4):283–6.

27. Ilizarov GA. Clinical application of the tension-stress effect for limb lengthening. Clin Orthop Relat Res 1990;250:8–26.

28. Matev IB. Thumb reconstruction in children through metacarpal lengthening. Plast Reconstr Surg 1979; 64(5):665–9.

29. Matev IB. Thumb reconstruction through metacarpal bone lengthening. J Hand Surg Am 1980;5(5):482–7.

30. Moy OJ, Peimer CA, Sherwin FS. Reconstruction of traumatic or congenital amputation of the thumb by distraction-lengthening. Hand Clin 1992;8(1):57–62.

31. Matev I. Thumb metacarpal lengthening. Tech Hand Up Extrem Surg 2003;7(4):157–63.

32. Azari K. Thumb reconstruction. In: Wolfe SW, Pederson WC, Kozin SH, et al, editors. Green's operative hand surgery. Elsevier; 2016.

33. Doi K, Hattori S, Kawai S, et al. New procedure on making a thumb–one-stage reconstruction with free neurovascular flap and iliac bone graft. J Hand Surg Am 1981;6(4):346–50.

34. Sabapathy SR, Venkatramani H, Bharathi RR. Functional evaluation of a great toe transfer and the osteoplastic technique for thumb reconstruction in the same individual. J Hand Surg Br 2003;28(5):405–8.

35. Morrison WA, O'Brien BM, MacLeod AM. Thumb reconstruction with a free neurovascular wrap-around flap from the big toe. J Hand Surg Am 1980;5(6):575–83.

36. Lee KS, Chae IJ, Hahn SB. Thumb reconstruction with a free neurovascular wrap-around flap from the big toe: long-term follow-up of thirty cases. Microsurgery 1995;16(10):692–7.

37. Wei FC, Chen HC, Chuang DC, et al. Second toe wrap-around flap. Plast Reconstr Surg 1991;88(5):837–43.

38. Nicoladoni C. Daumenplastik. Wien Klin Wochenschr 1897;28:663–6.

39. Cobbett JR. Free digital transfer. Report of a case of transfer of a great toe to replace an amputated thumb. J Bone Joint Surg Br 1969;51(4):677–9.

40. Replantation surgery surgery in China. Report of the American replantation mission to China. Plast Reconstr Surg 1973;52(5):476–89.

41. Gilbert A. Composite tissue transfer from the foot: anatomic basis and surgical technique. In: Symposium on Micro-surgery. Philadelphia, PA: CV Mosby Co; 1976. p. 1674–705.

42. Upton J. Direct visualization of arterial anatomy during toe harvest dissections: clinical and radiological correlations. Plast Reconstr Surg 1998;102(6):1988–92.

43. Gabrielli C, Olave E. Origins of the dorsal metatarsal arteries in humans. Scand J Plast ReConstr Surg Hand Surg 2002;36(4):221–5.

44. Hou Z, Zou J, Wang Z, et al. Anatomical classification of the first dorsal metatarsal artery and its clinical

application. Plast Reconstr Surg 2013;132(6):1028e–39e.

45. Steichen JB, Weiss AP. Reconstruction of traumatic absence of the thumb by microvascular free tissue transfer from the foot. Hand Clin 1992;8(1):17–32.

46. Buncke GM. Great toe to thumb transplantation. In: Tran TA, Panthaki ZJ, Hoballah JJ, et al, editors. Operative dictations in plastic and reconstructive surgery. Switzerland: Springer; 2017.

47. Robbins F, Reece T. Hand rehabilitation after great toe transfer for thumb reconstruction. Arch Phys Med Rehabil 1985;66(2):109–12.

48. Wei FC, Chen HC, Chuang CC, et al. Reconstruction of the thumb with a trimmed-toe transfer technique. Plast Reconstr Surg 1988;82(3):506–15.

49. Lin PY, Sebastin SJ, Ono S, et al. A systematic review of outcomes of toe-to-thumb transfers for isolated traumatic thumb amputation. Hand (N Y) 2011;6(3):235–43.

50. Troisi L, Mazzocconi L, Mastroiacovo A, et al. Beauty and function: the use of trimmed great toe in thumb and finger reconstruction. Plast Reconstr Surg Glob Open 2022;10(9):e4540.

51. Gordon L. Toe-to-thumb transplantation, . Operative hand surgery. New York Edinburgh: Churchill Livingstone; 1993. p. 1253–82.

52. Kim HS, Lee DC, Kim JS, et al. Donor-site morbidity after partial second toe pulp free flap for fingertip reconstruction. Arch Plast Surg 2016;43(1):66–70.

53. Tsai TM, McCabe S, Beatty ME. Second toe transfer for thumb reconstruction in multiple digit amputations including thumb and basal joint. Microsurgery 1987;8(3):146–53.

54. Lutz BS, Wei FC. Basic principles on toe-to-hand transplantation. Chang Gung Med J 2002;25(9):568–76.

55. Wei FC, Chen HC, Chuang CC, et al. Microsurgical thumb reconstruction with toe transfer: selection of various techniques. Plast Reconstr Surg 1994; 93(2):345–51. ; discussion 352-7.

56. Zhao J, Tien HY, Abdullah S, et al. Aesthetic refinements in second toe-to-thumb transfer surgery. Plast Reconstr Surg 2010;126(6):2052–9.

57. Lin CH, Lo S, Lin CH, et al. Opponensplasty provides predictable opposable tripod pinch in toe transfer for proximal thumb ray defect reconstruction. Plast Reconstr Surg 2012;130(6):810e–8e.

58. Harashina T. Analysis of 200 free flaps. Br J Plast Surg 1988;41(1):33–6.

59. Haughey BH, Wilson E, Kluwe L, et al. Free flap reconstruction of the head and neck: analysis of 241 cases. Otolaryngol Head Neck Surg 2001; 125(1):10–7.

60. Khouri RK, Shaw WW. Reconstruction of the lower extremity with microvascular free flaps: a 10-year experience with 304 consecutive cases. J Trauma 1989;29(8):1086–94.

61. Lin YT, Su ST, Lo S, et al. Risk factors for reexploration in toe-to-hand transfer: a multivariate analysis of 363 cases. Plast Reconstr Surg 2015;135(2):501–6.

62. Sosin M, Lin CH, Steinberg J, et al. Functional donor site morbidity after vascularized toe transfer procedures: a review of the literature and biomechanical consideration for surgical site selection. Ann Plast Surg 2016;76(6):735–42.

63. Maloney CT Jr, DeJesus R, Dellon AL. Painful foot neuromas after toe-to-thumb transfer. J Hand Surg Am 2005;30(1):105–10.

64. Chung KC, Wei FC. An outcome study of thumb reconstruction using microvascular toe transfer. J Hand Surg Am 2000;25(4):651–8.

65. Shaffrey EC, Moura SP, Attaluri PK, et al. Forty-year follow-up after great toe-to-thumb transfer: a literature review. J Hand Surg Glob Online 2023;5(3): 375–8.

66. Strickland JW, Kleinman WB. Thumb reconstruction. In: Green DP, editor. Operative hand surgery. New York: Elsevier-Health Sciences Division; 1993. p. 2043–156.

67. De Almeida YK, Athlani L, Piessat C, et al. Pollicization in the treatment of congenital severe hypoplasia and aplasia of the thumb: a systematic review. Hand Surg Rehabil 2022;41(1):22–30.

68. Kozin SH. Pollicization: the concept, technical details, and outcome. Clin Orthop Surg 2012;4(1): 18–35.

69. Chahine F, Bakhach JY. Pollicization. In: Tran TA, Panthaki ZJ, Hoballah JJ, et al, editors. Operative dictations in plastic and reconstructive surgery. Switzerland: Springer; 2017.

70. Brunelli GA, Brunelli GR. Reconstruction of traumatic absence of the thumb in the adult by pollicization. Hand Clin 1992;8(1):41–55.

71. Foucher G, Medlna J, Navarro R. Pollicization of damaged fingers. Tech Hand Up Extrem Surg 2000; 4(4):244–50.

72. Ishida O, Taniguchi Y, Sunagawa T, et al. Pollicization of the index finger for traumatic thumb amputation. Plast Reconstr Surg 2006;117(3):909–14.

73. Nikkhah D, Martin N, Pickford M. Paediatric toe-to-hand transfer: an assessment of outcomes from a single unit. J Hand Surg Eur 2016;41(3):281–94.

74. Kollitz KM, Tomhave W, Van Heest AE, et al. Change in hand function and dexterity with age after index pollicization for congenital thumb hypoplasia. Plast Reconstr Surg 2018;141(3):691–700.

75. Pillet J, Didierjean-Pillet A. Aesthetic hand prosthesis: gadget or therapy? presentation of a new classification. J Hand Surg Br 2001;26(6):523–8.

76. Li Y, Kulbacka-Ortiz K, Caine-Winterberger K, et al. Thumb amputations treated with osseointegrated percutaneous prostheses with up to 25 years of follow-up. J Am Acad Orthop Surg Glob Res Rev 2019;3(1):e097.

Pollicization and Pediatric Thumb Reconstruction

Brian W. Starr, MD[a,b,*], Kevin J. Little, MD[b,c]

KEYWORDS

- Pediatric thumb • Pollicization • Thumb reconstruction

KEY POINTS

- Pollicization is an elegant operation used for thumb reconstruction when the thumb is severely deficient or absent secondary to congenital anomalies or trauma.
- Classic indications include Blauth type IIIB, type IV, and type V thumb hypoplasia and traumatic loss of the thumb to the level of the basilar joint. Additional congenital indications include macrodactyly, multifingered hand, and ulnar dimelia.
- A thoughtful, stepwise approach coupled with meticulous surgical technique are critical to surgical success.
- Pediatric patients achieve superior outcomes and benefit from a greater capacity for cortical plasticity and motor relearning.

INTRODUCTION

In the words of John Napier, "The hand without a thumb is at worst nothing but an animated fish slice and at best a pair of forceps whose points don't meet properly."[1] Adrian Flatt later translated Napier's original British description to American English, replacing the word *fish slice* with *spatula*.[1,2] In either case, the role of the thumb as an integral part of the hand cannot be misinterpreted. In children, the absent or deficient thumb is most often the result of congenital hypoplasia. Alternatively, this can also occur secondary to trauma or a myriad of conditions, including macrodactyly, multifingered hand, and ulnar dimelia.[3,4]

Pollicization is an elegant operation that transforms an ordinary digit into an opposable thumb. The first account of thumb reconstruction using a pedicled digit can be traced back to Guermonprez in 1885.[5] The initial technique relied on the middle finger for reconstruction of traumatic thumb defects. Following the Second World War, in 1949,

Gosset took a leap forward by instead transferring the index finger into the thumb position.[5] Buck-Gramcko subsequently published his extensive study detailing over 400 cases of index pollicization, thus popularizing the technique that surgeons are familiar with today.[6] Over the last century, the operation has undergone refinements and modifications by many pioneers in the field of hand surgery.

INDICATIONS AND CONSIDERATIONS

Though pollicization is versatile enough to be used in a wide array of clinical scenarios, the most common indication, by modern accounts, is for the treatment of congenital thumb hypoplasia. Specifically, pollicization is the operation of choice for reconstructing a thumb with absent or unstable carpometacarpal (CMC) joint (Blauth types IIIB, IV, and V). Flatt and Kozin advocate for pollicization if the thumb is smaller than the small finger, regardless of CMC joint stability. Dr Kozin asserts that the

[a] Division of Pediatric Plastic Surgery, Department of Surgery, Cincinnati Children's Hospital Medical Center, 3333 Burnet Avenue, ML 2020, Cincinnati, OH 45229, USA; [b] University of Cincinnati College of Medicine, 3230 Eden Avenue, Cincinnati, OH 45267, USA; [c] Division of Pediatric Orthopedic Surgery, Department of Orthopedic Surgery, Cincinnati Children's Hospital Medical Center, 3333 Burnet Avenue, ML 2017, Cincinnati, OH 45229, USA
* Corresponding author.
E-mail address: Brian.starr@cchmc.org

Clin Plastic Surg 51 (2024) 575–582
https://doi.org/10.1016/j.cps.2024.04.002
0094-1298/24/© 2024 Elsevier Inc. All rights are reserved, including those for text and data mining, AI training, and similar technologies.

functional outcome of reconstructing a diminutive thumb with stable CMC joint "will pale in comparison" to a pollicized "normal" index finger.[3] Additional indications for pollicization in the pediatric patient include triphalangeal thumb (5 fingered hand), ulnar dimelia (mirror hand), and absent thumb in ulnar dysplasia (ulnar club hand). In setting of trauma, thumb amputation at the level of the CMC joint is an ideal indication. If the CMC joint is preserved, pollicization becomes less critical, and reconstructive options are expanded to include techniques including vascularized toe transfer and metacarpal lengthening.

Meticulous surgical technique is a prerequisite for successful pollicization. However, successful outcomes also rely on cortical plasticity and a propensity for motor relearning that are inherent to pediatric patients. Cortical plasticity is defined by the brain's ability to adapt previously inactive neural connections. New afferent pathways develop from neighboring cortical and/or subcortical regions. Using noninvasive brain stimulation techniques on individuals aged 19 to 81 years, Freitas and colleagues[7] objectively demonstrated that the mechanisms attributed to cortical plasticity decrease in efficiency over time. Pediatric patients are exceptionally well equipped for cortical adaptation and regeneration, as evidenced by the reversible massive cortical reorganization seen in 6 year old Zion Harvey, following bilateral hand allotransplantation.[8] Furthermore, functional MRI research indicates that motor reorganization is influenced by experience and training and continues to progress over time.[9] Though there are no studies specifically examining the neural reorganization that takes place following pollicization, existing neuroscience literature underscores the concept that pediatric patients are ideally suited to achieve optimal outcomes.

POLLICIZATION TECHNIQUE

A methodical, stepwise approach is used to ensure safe, reproducible–and teachable–technique. Note that procedure nuances may require adaptation in accordance with variations in clinical presentation and underlying anatomy.

1. Skin incision: The design must be thoughtful to allow excellent exposure and transposition of the index finger, while also providing an end-result with a deep first webspace. Various flap and incision design techniques exist. The authors follow the technique as described by Kozin, Ezaki, and Carter, which facilitates transfer and optimal use of glabrous skin to reconstruct the first webspace.[3] This approach also improves the overall esthetics of the reconstructed thumb, lest the final product look too much like a finger.

Mirror-image curved incisions are designed along the volar and dorsal aspect of the index finger, with the proximal apex of each incision at the midaxis of the radial and ulnar metacarpophalangeal (MCP) joint. The dorsal fish mouth is designed more proximally, with the volar incision placed distally approaching the level of the PIP joint crease (**Fig. 1**). From the radial MCP joint apex, a curved incision is drawn along the palmar-radial border of the hand, approaching the index CMC joint. If a hypoplastic thumb is being removed, care must be taken to preserve adequate skin, while incorporating the resection into the planned incision, typically with an elliptical incision around the base.

2. Isolation of neurovascular bundles: Under loupe magnification, the palmar-radial incision is made, and the radial neurovascular bundle is identified. A hypoplastic thumb will typically have a connection to the radial digital artery, which helps in identifying this structure, which is often hypoplastic or even absent. Modest exsanguination technique prior to tourniquet inflation will aid in vessel identification. Palmar dissection proceeds ulnarly to isolate the common digital neurovascular bundle to index/long finger (**Fig. 2**).

3. Neurolysis: The proper digital nerve to the radial long finger and ulnar index finger must be identified and meticulously separated out via intrafascicular dissection proximally. Failure to perform this step will impede tension-free transposition.

4. Vessel ligation: The proper digital artery to the radial aspect of the long finger is identified and ligated. Whether the decision is to use vessel clips or silk ties, the authors advise using ligating material that remains easily visible and serves as a clear reminder of vessel location.

5. Pulley release: The A1 and A2 pulleys to the index finger are incised (**Fig. 3**).[10] Failure to perform adequate pulley release will lead to buckling of the flexor tendons when the digit is transposed and shortened.

6. Elevate dorsal skin flap: Performing this step in a somewhat delayed manner allows for filling and vasodilation of the dorsal vein while the surgeon works palmarly. This aids in visualization during dorsal flap elevation. Preservation of dorsal veins by means of meticulous dissection is paramount to avoiding venous congestion and potential compromise of the transposed digit (**Fig. 4**). This is done by meticulous dissection proximally and distally immediately below the dermis a

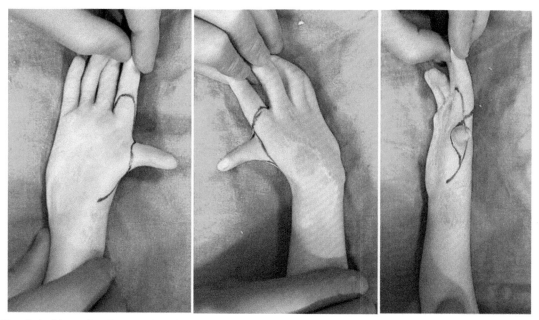

Fig. 1. Incision planning. Patient is a 6 year old boy undergoing pollicization 4 years following wrist centralization.

well as deeper between the veins and the extensor tendons to fully isolate and mobilize the veins to allow for transposition without stretching, kinking, or congesting the venous outflow.

7. Dissection of extrinsic tendons: Extensor digitorum and extensor indices tendons (when both are present) are dissected free from the second metacarpal and surrounding tissue to ensure a straight line of pull. Distally, the extrinsic extensors must be isolated from the intrinsic muscles. No additional dissection of the flexor tendons is indicated. Shortening of the extrinsic flexor and extensor tendons is

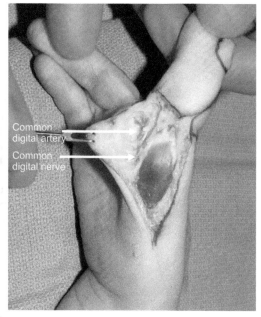

Fig. 2. Exposure of common digital artery to index/long finger and common digital nerve to index finger.

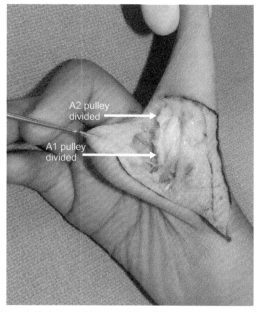

Fig. 3. Release of A1 and A2 pulleys. A2 is not critical to preserve, and release facilitates transposition.

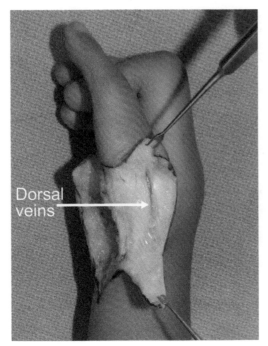

Fig. 4. Dorsal venous outflow must be preserved to avoid compromise of the transposed digit.

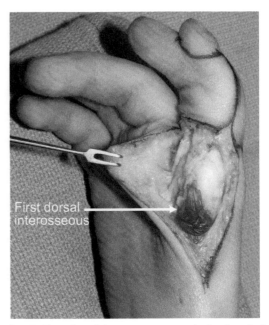

Fig. 5. First dorsal interosseous muscle is dissected distally and released prior to transfer into the radial lateral band.

not indicated. Some authors advise shortening the extensor tendons by Utilizing extensor indices proprius (EIP) as a new extensor pollicis longus (EPL) and extensor digitorum communis (EDC) to index as a new abductor pollicis longus (APL) tendon, if both tendons are present.

8. Dissection of intrinsic muscles: The first dorsal and first palmar interosseous muscles are identified. Sharp dissection proceeds distally to the level of the extensor hood insertion. Interossei are sharply elevated off the index metacarpal in a supraperiosteal plane (Fig. 5). Distally, care is taken to avoid injury to the index radial collateral ligament while harvesting a small strip of extensor hood with the dissection. Failure to preserve length on the distal interossei will make readvancement and muscle inset more challenging.

9. Tag lateral bands: The radial and ulnar lateral bands are identified and tagged to facilitate ease of inset in the final steps of the procedure (Fig. 6). Failure to tag lateral bands prior to osteotomy will make identification and orientation more challenging (Fig. 7).

10. Osteotomy: A Beaver blade or fine oscillating saw is used to perform distal osteotomy through the physis. The intermetacarpal ligament is incised, and the proximal index metacarpal is cut at the metaphyseal flare with a bone cutter allowing the metacarpal diaphysis

to be removed (see Fig. 7A and B). Failure to perform epiphysiodesis will result in excessive growth of the pollicized digit.

11. Reposition index MCP joint: In contrast to the index finger MCP joint, the normal anatomy of

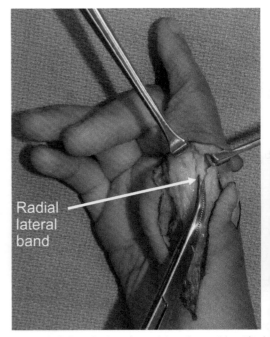

Fig. 6. Radial and ulnar lateral bands are identified and tagged.

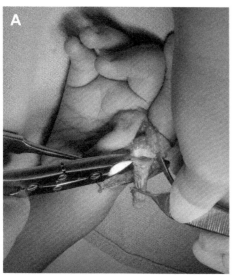
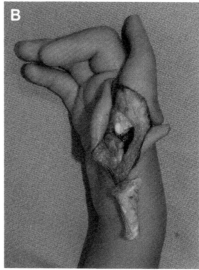

Fig. 7. (*A* and *B*) Distal osteotomy cut is made through the physis. Proximally, the metacarpal is cut at the metaphyseal flare with a bone cutter allowing the metacarpal diaphysis to be removed.

the thumb CMC joint does not permit hyperextension. Prior to transposition, permanent suture is used to secure the metacarpal epiphysis to the dorsal capsule and fix the index MCP joint in hyperextension.

12. Pinning of transposed digit: The shortened index metacarpal is transposed and placed into 20° radial abduction and 35° palmar abduction and 100° to 120° of pronation prior to retrograde pinning with a 0.045 inch Kirchner wire (**Fig. 8**).

13. Tendon transfers: The first dorsal interosseous tendon is secured to the previously tagged radial lateral band (reconstructed abductor). The first palmar interosseus is secured to the previously tagged ulnar lateral band (reconstructed adductor).

14. Flap inset: The tourniquet is deflated, hemostasis is confirmed, and flaps are inset. Pink, healthy perfusion of the thumb is confirmed following skin flap inset (**Fig. 9**).

15. Dressing: The novel thumb is protected with a well-padded, above-elbow cast. The elbow should be positioned in 100° of flexion with a mold to preempt unintended removal. The patient is admitted overnight for pain control, elevation, and monitoring.

OUTCOMES

Abundant retrospective studies have documented positive outcomes following pollicization, namely with regards to improved overall function and appearance (**Fig. 10**).[11–18] However, it would be naïve to think that pollicization can reconstruct a "normal" thumb. Postoperative dexterity, range

of motion, grip and pinch strength are consistently reduced compared to unaffected controls.[14,18–20] Outcomes are dependent on the baseline functional capacity of the digit to be transferred, as well as the status of existing intrinsic musculature. Better results are seen in younger patients with isolated congenital thumb hypoplasia.[19]

Objective interpretation of historical outcomes remains somewhat elusive, in part due to variability

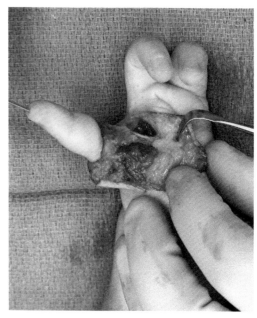

Fig. 8. The transposed digit is pinned in 20° radial abduction and 35° palmar abduction and 100° to 120° of pronation. Note that there is no kinking or tension on the neurovascular bundle.

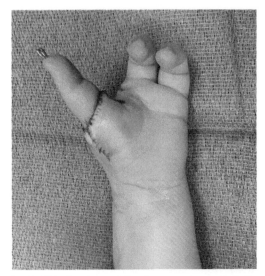

Fig. 9. Skin flap inset following tourniquet deflation demonstrating a well-perfused, pink digit. The transposed digit must be critically assessed for any evidence of vascular compromise or venous congestion.

of surgeon technique, patient population, and lack of a standardized assessment tool.[21] Kollitz and colleagues[22] recently found the novel thumb grasp and pinch assessment to be the only functional measure to correlate with overall patient and family satisfaction following pollicization. Compared to unaffected norms, estimates of grip and pinch strength vary widely and are largely dependent on the severity of concomitant radial longitudinal deficiency.[23–25] In relatively mild cases, grip and pinch strength have been reported as high as 76% and 56% of the contralateral side, respectively, though these measurements are often far weaker.[24,26] In a retrospective review of 28 cases, Manske reported that mean grip strength and

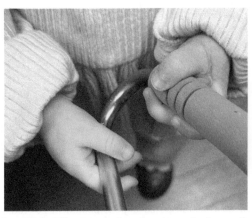

Fig. 10. Excellent early functional result, 3 months postop, in a 2 year old patient with history of bilateral ulnar longitudinal dysplasia.

lateral, tripod, and tip pinch were reduced nearly 80% compared to standard measurements.[16]

Despite reduced strength and range of motion, De Kraker and colleagues[14] reported high satisfaction among patients and parents regarding surgical outcome. Furthermore, in a retrospective review of 23 patients with 29 affected thumbs who underwent pollicization, Kollitz and colleagues[27] found that metrics of dexterity and strength increased each year. Notably, the authors acknowledged that webspace did not increase with age and that attentive positioning must be performed at the time of initial surgery.

COMPLICATIONS

The stepwise approach to pollicization is well established and delivers predictable outcomes with experience, sound surgical technique, and attention to detail. Nevertheless, there are numerous shortcomings that the surgeon must understand and must communicate clearly to the family.

In 2009, Goldfarb and colleagues published a retrospective review of Dr Manske's experience chronicling 73 pollicizations over 30 years, specifically examining complications and shortcomings. In the early postop period, the authors reported an 11% complication rate, including marginal skin necrosis in 5.5% of patients, venous congestion in 4.1%, and infection in 1.4%. One of the 3 digits that suffered from venous congestion was not able to be salvaged. Dorsal veins are fragile and inherently prone to kinking with the transposition. Goldfarb and colleagues[28] stress the importance of vigilant postoperative monitoring and a low threshold to return to the operating room for exploration in the setting of impaired venous outflow.

In addition, the authors report suboptimal outcomes in 11% of patients, related to 7 cases of scar contracture and 1 case of redundant skin. Scar contracture required surgical release in 2 patients, who were effectively treated with Z-plasty. Furthermore, 26% of patients suffered from poor opposition postoperatively. Seventeen of 19 (89%) of these patients improved following abductor digiti minimi opponensplasty, performed at a mean of 26 months following pollicization. Two patients required additional FDS transfer to adequately augment opposition function. Overall, 51% (37 out of 73) of digits required additional surgery following the initial pollicization operation.[28]

ALTERNATIVES

As previously discussed, pollicization is an ideal operation in type IIIB or type IV thumb hypoplasia where intrinsic and extrinsic motors are weak or absent and the basilar joint is grossly unstable. However, the surgical approach and preoperative discussion must also carefully consider the specific needs of the individual patient and family. The authors wholeheartedly agree with Drs Flatt, Kozin, and many others that a functional, well-positioned index finger serves as the best replacement for a severely deficient thumb. However, there are an array of scenarios—most often related to cultural norms—where index pollicization with hypoplastic thumb ablation is not acceptable. In these scenarios, the surgeon must be candid about treatment goals as well as limitations.

Shibata and colleagues initially described vascularized toe joint transfer for type IIIB hypoplastic thumb reconstruction, a method that was subsequently popularized by Tong and colleagues and Dautel.[29–31] This approach aims to reconstruct a stable thumb, in opposition, by transferring a vascularized metatarsophalangeal joint from the second toe.[30,31] Alternative, nonvascularized approaches that rely on nonvascularized bone graft and CMC joint arthrodesis fail to address the challenge of reconstruction in a growing child.[32] Free tissue transfer obviates this problem by incorporating the viable epiphyseal plate of the metatarsal bone and proximal phalanx in the transfer. This technique preserves the potential for future growth.

Luangjarmekorn and colleagues[33] elucidate key indications and contraindications for vascularized second toe joint transfer in their detailed technique article. Indications include (1) type IIIB and type IV thumbs; (2) a patient and family who decline hypoplastic thumb ablation and index pollicization; (3) a patient and family who value a 5 digit hand over a 4 digit hand; and (4) a patient and family who are willing to accept a stiff thumb held in opposition. Conversely, contraindications for this procedure are (1) a patient and family who prioritize maximum motion in the thumb's CMC and MCP joints; (2) patient and family who are unwilling to tolerate foot morbidity; (3) a patient who is unable to endure extended operative times (expect at least 6 hours); and (4) those who are unwilling to accept the risk of flap loss and potential necrosis of the hypoplastic thumb.

CLINICS CARE POINTS

- Index finger pollicization is the operation of. Pollicization does not reconstruct a "normal" thumb.
- A methodical, stepwise, meticulous approach is essential. Omitting steps will preclude

effective transposition, or worse, leading to the kinking of neurovascular structures.

- Secondary operations are common. Hand therapy and long-term follow-up are instrumental to determine additional functional needs and to help guide intervention.

DISCLOSURES

The authors have no conflicts of interest to disclose.

REFERENCES

1. Napier J. hands, rev ed. princeton, NJ: Princeton university press, 1993:55.
2. Our Thumbs_Flatt_BUMC proceedings 2002.
3. Kozin SH. Pollicization: the concept, technical details, and outcome. Clin Orthop Surg 2012;4(1): 18–35.
4. Canizares MF, Feldman L, Miller PE, et al. Pollicization of the index finger in the United States: early readmission and complications. J Hand Surg 2019; 44(9):795.e1–8.
5. Littler JW, strickland JW. On making a thumb: a century of surgical effort. In: Weinzweig N, weinzweig J, editors. The mutilated hand. philadelphia, pensylvania. Philadelphia, PA: Elsevier Mosby; 2005. p. 99–111.
6. Buck-Gramcko D. Pollicization of the index finger. method and results in aplasia and hypoplasia of the thumb. J Bone Joint Surg Am 1971;53(8): 1605–17.
7. Freitas C, Perez J, Knobel M, et al. Changes in cortical plasticity across the lifespan. Front Aging Neurosci 2011;3:5.
8. Gaetz W, Kessler SK, Roberts TPL, et al. Massive cortical reorganization is reversible following bilateral transplants of the hands: evidence from the first successful bilateral pediatric hand transplant patient. Ann Clin Transl Neurol 2017;5(1):92–7.
9. Chen R, Anastakis DJ, Haywood CT, et al. Plasticity of the human motor system following muscle reconstruction: a magnetic stimulation and functional magnetic resonance imaging study. Clin Neurophysiol 2003;114(12):2434–46.
10. Carter PR, Ezaki M, Oishi S. Index pollicization: an evolution of ideas and techniques from a paediatric orthopaedic institution. J Hand Surg Eur 2022; 47(10):1004.
11. Aliu O, Netscher DT, Staines KG, et al. A 5-year interval evaluation of function after pollicization for congenital thumb aplasia using multiple outcome measures. Plast Reconstr Surg 2008;122(1):198–205.
12. Goldfarb CA, Deardorff V, Chia B, et al. Objective features and aesthetic outcome of pollicized digits

compared with normal thumbs. J Hand Surg Am 2007;32(7):1031–6.

13. Staines KG, Majzoub R, Thornby J, et al. Functional outcome for children with thumb aplasia undergoing pollicization. Plast Reconstr Surg 2005;116(5): 1314–5.

14. de Kraker M, Selles RW, van Vooren J, et al. Outcome after pollicization: comparison of patients with mild and severe longitudinal radial deficiency. Plast Reconstr Surg 2013;131(4):544e–51e.

15. Kozin SH, Weiss AA, Webber JB, et al. Index finger pollicization for congenital aplasia or hypoplasia of the thumb. J Hand Surg Am 1992;17(5):880–4.

16. Manske PR, Rotman MB, Dailey LA. Long-term functional results after pollicization for the congenitally deficient thumb. J Hand Surg Am 1992;17(6):1064–72.

17. Sykes PJ, Chandraprakasam T, Percival NJ. Pollicisation of the index finger in congenital anomalies. A retrospective analysis. J Hand Surg Br 1991; 16(2):144–7.

18. Netscher DT, Aliu O, Sandvall BK, et al. Functional outcomes of children with index pollicizations for thumb deficiency. J Hand Surg Am 2013;38(2):250–7.

19. Lightdale-Miric N, Mueske NM, Lawrence EL, et al. Long term functional outcomes after early childhood pollicization. J Hand Ther 2014;28(2):158.

20. Manske PR, McCarroll HR. Reconstruction of the congenitally deficient thumb. Hand Clin 1992;8(1): 177–96. Available at: https://www.sciencedirect.com/science/article/pii/S0749071221007010.

21. Zlotolow DA, Tosti R, Ashworth S, et al. Developing a pollicization outcomes measure. J Hand Surg Am 2014;39(9):1784–91.

22. Kollitz KM, Tomhave WA, Van Heest AE, et al. A new, direct measure of thumb use in children after index pollicization for congenital thumb hypoplasia. J Hand Surg Am 2018;43(11):978–86.e1.

23. Percival NJ, Sykes PJ, Chandraprakasam T. A method of assessment of pollicisation. J Hand Surg Br 1991;16(2):141–3.

24. Roper BA, Turnbull TJ. Functional assessment after pollicisation. J Hand Surg Br 1986;11(3):399–403.

25. Sletten IN, Røkkum M, Winge MI. Outcome after pollicization for congenital thumb deficiency: a cohort study of cases in a single unit, 1987 to 2016. J Hand Surg 2022;47(5):479.

26. Vekris MD, Beris AE, Lykissas MG, et al. Index finger pollicization in the treatment of congenitally deficient thumb. Ann Plast Surg 2011;66(2):137–42.

27. Kollitz K, Tomhave W, Van Heest A, et al. Change in hand function and dexterity with age after index pollicization for congenital thumb hypoplasia. Plast Reconstr Surg 2018;141(3):691–700. Available at: http://ovidsp.ovid.com/ovidweb.cgi?T=JS&NEWS=n&CSC=Y&PAGE=fulltext&D=ovft&AN=00006534-201803000-00022.

28. Goldfarb CA, Monroe E, Steffen J, et al. Incidence and treatment of complications, suboptimal outcomes, and functional deficiencies after pollicization. J Hand Surg Am 2009;34(7):1291–7.

29. Shibata M, Yoshizu T, Seki T, et al. Reconstruction of a congenital hypoplastic thumb with use of a free vascularized metatarsophalangeal joint. J Bone Joint Surg Am 1998;80(10):1469–76.

30. Tong D, Wu L, Li P, et al. Reversed vascularized second metatarsal flap for reconstruction of manske type IIIB and IV thumb hypoplasia with reduced donor site morbidity. Chin Med J (Engl) 2019; 132(21):2565–71.

31. Dautel G. Vascularized toe joint transfers to the hand for PIP or MCP reconstruction. Hand Surg Rehabil 2018;37(6):329–36.

32. Tajima T. Classification of thumb hypoplasia. Hand Clin 1985;1(3):577–94.

33. Luangjarmekorn P, Pongernnak N, Kitidumrongsook P. Vascularized Toe Joint Transfer for Hypoplastic Thumb Type IV. Tech Hand Up Extrem. Surg 2021;25(4): 226–34.

Current and Future Directions for Upper Extremity Amputations

Comparisons Between Regenerative Peripheral Nerve Interface and Targeted Muscle Reinnervation Surgeries

Christine S.W. Best, MD[a], Theodore A. Kung, MD[b],*

KEYWORDS

- Amputation • Neuropathic pain • Phantom pain • Residual limb pain • Neuroma
- Regenerative peripheral nerve interface surgery • Targeted muscle reinnervation surgery
- Prosthetic control

KEY POINTS

- Pain from symptomatic neuromas is a substantial cause of morbidity in people with upper extremity amputation.
- Regenerative peripheral nerve interface (RPNI) surgery and targeted muscle reinnervation (TMR) surgery are effective in reducing chronic postamputation pain including residual limb pain and phantom pain.
- RPNI and TMR surgeries have the potential to facilitate control of advanced upper extremity prosthetic limbs.
- The main difference between RPNI and TMR surgeries is the surgical technique; however, both strategies rely on physiologic processes such as nerve regeneration and muscle reinnervation.

INTRODUCTION

Greater than 1 million extremity amputations are performed worldwide every year,[1] with major upper extremity amputation less commonly performed than major lower extremity amputation.[2] Upper extremity amputations are mostly secondary to traumatic injury (approximately 80%), although limb amputation may also be indicated to treat malignancy, vascular complications, infection, congenital deformity, or to manage refractory pain. Amputations are named based on the level at which they are performed, and in the upper extremity these levels from proximal to distal are forequarter, shoulder disarticulation, transhumeral, elbow disarticulation, transradial, wrist disarticulation, transcarpal, transmetacarpal, and transphalangeal/digital. Digital amputations account for

[a] Department of Surgery, Section of Plastic Surgery, University of Michigan, 1500 East Medical Center Drive, 2110 Taubman Center, SPC 5346, Ann Arbor, MI 48109-5346, USA; [b] Department of Surgery, Section of Plastic Surgery, University of Michigan, 1500 East Medical Center Drive, 2130 Taubman Center, Ann Arbor, MI 48109-5231, USA
* Corresponding author. Section of Plastic Surgery, 1500 East Medical Center Drive, 2130 Taubman Center, Ann Arbor, MI 48109-5231.
E-mail address: thekung@med.umich.edu

Clin Plastic Surg 51 (2024) 583–592
https://doi.org/10.1016/j.cps.2024.05.001

approximately 80% of all upper extremity amputations, while major upper extremity amputations (proximal to the wrist joint) account for approximately 8%.[3]

The prevalence of chronic pain after amputation varies between 10% and 76%[4–7] with increased risk in patients after traumatic amputation, transhumeral amputation, and forequarter amputation.[8] Chronic pain can be isolated to the residual limb itself (ie, residual limb pain) or as phantom limb pain. Neuropathic pain is caused by multiple cut peripheral nerves during upper extremity amputation, and thus, the prevention of painful neuromas is critically important to maximize the quality of life for these patients. Normally, after peripheral nerve transection, the nerve undergoes biologic processes including Wallerian degeneration, axonal sprouting, and muscle reinnervation if end organs are present.[9] However, in the setting of amputation, the end organs are missing and thus the cut peripheral nerves in the limb continue to sprout and regenerate aimlessly, leading to the formation of neuromas. The prevalence of symptomatic upper limb neuromas after amputation has been reported by some authors to be approximately 25%.[10,11] Symptomatic neuroma pain can be characterized by burning, aching, and tingling pain coupled with a positive Tinel's sign, defined as solicitation of neuropathic sensations with manual tapping along an injured nerve. Other studies have shown higher incidences of symptomatic neuromas of up to 50% to 70% after limb loss[10,12,13] and that neuromas are known to compromise prosthetic rehabilitation and diminish the quality of life.[14]

Many treatment modalities have been explored for symptomatic neuromas. Nonsurgical treatments include desensitization, biofeedback, anesthetic or chemical injections, topical anesthetics, pain catheters, and various pharmacologic agents. Surgical treatments for symptomatic neuromas include neuroma excision, nerve capping, excision with transposition into muscle or bone, and nerve grafting.[15–21] In addition to these management techniques, 2 newer surgical procedures have been introduced for the prevention and treatment of painful neuroma and postamputation pain: regenerative peripheral nerve interface (RPNI) surgery and targeted muscle reinnervation (TMR) surgery.

The critical goals after upper extremity amputation are to preserve length, minimize pain, and maintain or improve functional status. This article provides an overview of the use of RPNI and TMR surgeries as novel surgical strategies to help patients reduce postamputation pain and to optimize prosthetic rehabilitation after upper extremity amputation.

REGENERATIVE PERIPHERAL NERVE INTERFACE SURGERY

An RPNI is constructed by implanting the distal end of a transected peripheral nerve into a denervated autologous free skeletal muscle graft (Fig. 1). As the peripheral nerve regenerates, it readily reinnervates the denervated skeletal muscle graft and forms new neuromuscular junctions. The free skeletal muscle graft is known to also undergo a well-described process of degeneration followed by regeneration that occurs concurrently with nerve regeneration.[22–24] Initially, the RPNI technique was devised as a strategy to capture volitional motor command signals from peripheral nerves to control an advanced neuroprosthetic device. Reinnervation of the free skeletal muscle grafts enabled transduction of relatively small neural signals into high-amplitude electromyographic signals when an electrode was placed within the RPNI muscle. RPNI surgery can be performed on major upper extremity peripheral nerves (ie, radial, median, and ulnar) to amplify native efferent peripheral nerve signals to control a prosthetic device.[25,26] The process of successfully reinnervating these free skeletal muscle grafts also dramatically reduces the number of aimless axons present at the site of peripheral nerve regeneration. Therefore, it was subsequently discovered that RPNI surgery also had immense potential to prevent the formation of neuromas.[27] Importantly, RPNI surgery differs from the conventional approach of burying a free nerve end into an adjacent muscle belly; in this technique, the muscle fibers of the adjacent muscle remain innervated and, therefore, the regenerating axons of the cut peripheral nerve are not presented with denervated targets. Thus, a new neuroma will certainly form within the adjacent muscle belly. In contrast with RPNI surgery, the autologous free muscle graft provides ample denervated muscle fibers with which regenerating axons can connect to form new and functional neuromuscular junctions, thereby reducing the propensity of neuroma development.

Surgical Technique

Creating an RPNI is straightforward and can be performed on any transected peripheral nerve. First, the surgeon exposes the transected peripheral nerve end, and the nerve is freed from any attachments. If a neuroma is present at the end of the peripheral nerve, it is sharply excised, and the nerve is bread-loafed until healthy fascicles are visualized (Fig. 2). Interfascicular dissection can be performed with tenotomy scissors to separate and identify component fascicles as needed

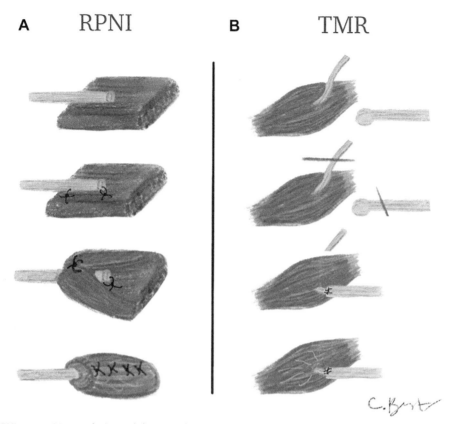

A RPNI   **B TMR**

Fig. 1. RPNI versus TMR technique. (A) RPNI: The transected peripheral nerve is implanted into the free muscle graft and secured with 2 tacking sutures, one in the distal end of the nerve epineurium into the middle of the muscle graft and one at the proximal end of the nerve. The entire muscle graft is wrapped longitudinally around the nerve and secured in place with sutures. (B) TMR: The peripheral nerve/neuroma is cut and the motor nerve is sacrificed. The transected peripheral nerve is coapted to the smaller sacrificed motor nerve with sutures at a level close to the denervated muscle. (*Courtesy of* Christine Best, MD.)

Often, robust bleeding will be encountered from the endogenous blood supply within the peripheral nerve, and this is controlled with careful bipolar cautery. Free skeletal muscle grafts are harvested locally from the amputation site (eg, brachioradialis), from the distal amputated limb if medically appropriate, or from any other remote skeletal muscle donor site (ie, vastus lateralis). The muscle graft can be harvested either individually or en bloc with scissors and then divided into approximately 30 mm long × 20 mm wide × 5 mm thick grafts (see **Fig. 2**). Harvest is done without cautery to avoid thermal injury to the free skeletal muscle grafts. The distal nerve or fascicle end is implanted into the center of a single free skeletal muscle graft using 6-0 polypropylene sutures to secure the epineurium to the muscle tissue. The muscle graft is then wrapped longitudinally around the nerve and sewn together using interrupted 6-0 polypropylene sutures (see **Fig. 2**). A well-vascularized pocket is then bluntly created and the RPNIs are positioned deep within the soft tissue closure.

Clinical Outcomes

Treating symptomatic neuromas after amputation is important to improve the quality of life for patients. Studies examining RPNI surgery efficacy in treating postamputation pain was initially motivated by encouraging feedback from patients during the rehabilitation course after limb amputation. One study demonstrated that RPNI surgery can help decrease residual limb pain from neuroma by 71% and reduce phantom limb pain by 53%.[27] In addition, patients reported high satisfaction levels and many reported using less opioid pain medications after RPNI surgery.[27] Another study demonstrated that patients who have prophylactic RPNI surgery at the time of amputation have significantly lower rates of phantom limb pain (51.1% vs 91.1%) as well as lower rates of symptomatic neuromas (0% vs 13.3%) on examination.[28] A prospective clinical trial examining the efficacy of RPNI surgery to treat symptomatic neuromas in major lower limb amputation patients

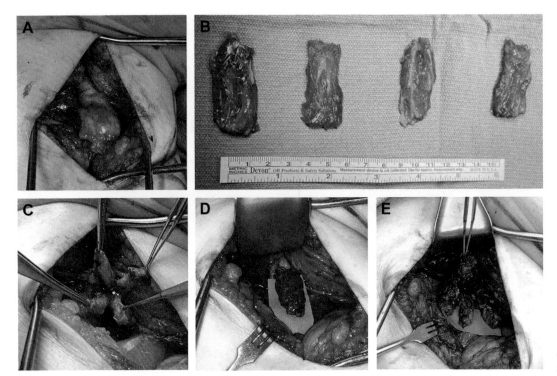

Fig. 2. Excision of neuroma and creation of fascicular RPNIs. (*A*) Neuroma is exposed and sharply transected en bloc to healthy-appearing nerve. (*B*) Harvest of autologous nonvascularized free skeletal muscle grafts (~30 mm long × 20 mm wide × 5 mm thick). (*C*) Interfascicular dissection into 4 distinct fascicles. (*D*) Creation of one RPNI by implanting nerve fascicle into free muscle graft. (*E*) All 4 RPNIs performed by securing nerve within separate skeletal muscle graft.

was completed in the fall of 2023. Analysis of patient-reported outcomes after RPNI surgery compared to preoperative assessment reveals significant differences in pain scores and quality in favor of RPNI intervention (Lee JC, Best CS, Hamill JB, et al. Regenerative Peripheral Nerve Interface (RPNI) Surgery for Treatment of Painful Neuroma in Lower Limb Amputations: One Year Outcomes. 2024). Furthermore, RPNI surgery was also significantly associated with better postoperative scores for psychosocial measurements for pain catastrophizing, anxiety, and depression. While this trial enrolled major lower limb amputation patients, the authors suggest that the findings can be extrapolated to upper extremity patients as well. With these encouraging experiences, RPNI surgery is also being studied prospectively in a variety of clinical settings, including hand and digit amputations as well as soft tissue tumor resections.

TARGETED MUSCLE REINNERVATION SURGERY

TMR surgery is a nerve transfer procedure designed to reroute transected peripheral nerves to nearby motor nerve branches (see **Fig. 1**).

Initially developed to enable myoelectric rehabilitation in upper extremity amputation patients, TMR has also been adapted for use in treating neuroma pain and phantom limb pain. In this operation, transected peripheral nerves are transferred to nearby motors nerves that are intentionally cut to denervate a patch of skeletal muscle for reinnervation. A nerve transfer is then performed to the cut motor nerve and the regenerating axons then reinnervate this purposefully denervated muscle (see **Fig. 1**). Importantly, like RPNI surgery, the fundamental processes that are involved with TMR surgery include nerve regeneration and muscle reinnervation. While several variations of TMR surgery have been described,[29] all share the common principle that muscle denervation is performed in order to allow for subsequent muscle reinnervation. From a prosthetic rehabilitation standpoint, once reinnervation has occurred in the muscle, surface electromyography electrodes can be placed to detect these rerouted motor commands to achieve prosthetic control.[30,31]

Surgical Technique

TMR surgery requires rerouting a transected peripheral nerve end to a nearby sacrificed motor

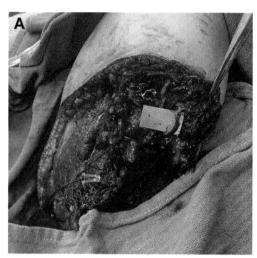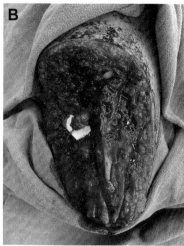

Fig. 3. Creation of TMR. (*A*) Coaptation of peripheral nerve and small sacrificed motor nerve. (*B*) Coaptation of larger caliber donor nerve to a smaller caliber recipient motor branch showing size mismatch.

nerve branch. Motor nerves innervating nearby muscles are identified using a handheld nerve stimulator and then divided. The peripheral nerve and the sacrificed motor nerve are then coapted together with 6-0 or 7-0 nonabsorbable sutures under loupe magnification (**Fig. 3**). Regional anesthesia is typically not used for TMR cases given the need to identify motor branches using handheld stimulation. Various nerve transfers have been described depending on the location of the amputation.[32,33] For example, for a shoulder disarticulation, the donor nerves include the musculocutaneous, median, ulnar, and radial nerves, with respective recipient motor nerves being the motor branch to the pectoral clavicular head, pectoral upper sternal head, pectoral lower sternal head, and the thoracodorsal nerve. For a transhumeral amputation, the donor nerves include the median, ulnar, and radial nerves, with respective recipient nerves being the musculocutaneous motor branch to biceps, musculocutaneous motor branch to brachialis, and radial motor branch to triceps. For a transradial amputation, the donor nerves include the median, ulnar, superficial branch of radial, lateral antebrachial cutaneous, and medial antebrachial cutaneous nerves, with recipient nerves being the anterior interosseous, ulnar motor branch, radial motor branch, median motor branch, and ulnar motor branch, respectively. For partial hand amputations, digital nerves can be connected to recipient motor branches of palmar/dorsal interosseous muscles.[32,34] In most cases, TMR surgery involves the transfer of a larger caliber donor nerve to a smaller caliber recipient motor branch and care must be taken to avoid large gaps in the nerve coaptation (see **Fig. 3**). Some authors describe the intussusception of the

smaller recipient motor nerve into the larger donor nerve with 1-2 polypropylene sutures, as well as making sure all parts of the operation are completed in a tension-free manner.[34] The greater the size mismatch, the more likely that there will be a neuroma-in-continuity that forms after TMR surgery[35–37]; however, some authors have not reported issues with the size mismatch.[38] Despite the limitation of neuromas-in-continuity, TMR surgery remains a proven strategy to improve postamputation pain. Some authors have proposed modification to the original TMR technique to address the issue of size mismatch, such as performing the coaptation within the denervated muscle belly or wrapping a free skeletal muscle graft around the coaptation site, which is a way to combine the principles of RPNI and TMR surgeries.[36,39]

Clinical Outcomes

TMR surgery has been shown to be a successful technique to treat chronic postamputation pain, including residual limb pain and phantom limb pain. In a randomized clinical trial involving upper and lower limb amputation patients evaluating TMR surgery versus conventional neurectomy, TMR surgery improved phantom limb pain with significantly better pain scores and trended toward improved residual limb pain postoperatively at 1 year.[38] A retrospective study also specifically showed that TMR surgery can be helpful to resolve and improve neuroma pain specifically in amputation patients.[40] TMR surgery has also been shown to be helpful in reducing the development and severity of residual limb pain and phantom limb pain when performed at the time of amputation, with significant improvement in patient-reported outcome scores compared to controls.[35,41] Additionally, another study showed that patients who underwent prophylactic TMR surgery at the time of amputation had decreased rates of neuroma formation compared to TMR surgery performed in a delayed manner (1.4% vs 18.8%), highlighting the role of TMR in the prevention of postamputation pain and prevention of neuroma.[42]

COMPLICATIONS AND LIMITATIONS: REGENERATIVE PERIPHERAL NERVE INTERFACE AND TARGETED MUSCLE REINNERVATION SURGERIES

Complications after RPNI and TMR surgeries largely relate to those expected after limb amputation, such as surgical site infection and delayed wound healing. Wound healing complications are most common as patients undergoing amputations frequently have other risk factors including diabetes, vascular disease, malnutrition, and/or trauma. Additionally, inadequate mitigation of postamputation pain and creation of new pain are also risks of the surgery.

Both RPNI and TMR surgeries have unique limitations and complication profiles. Successful RPNI surgery largely depends on the provision of a sufficient number of denervated muscle fibers for each regenerating peripheral nerve or fascicle. If the free skeletal muscle graft is too small, there will not be enough denervated muscle fiber targets for the regenerating axons, and therefore, a recurrent neuroma of variable size will form.[43] Conversely, because the survival of the free skeletal muscle graft is contingent on the physiologic processes of muscle regeneration and revascularization, if an excessive amount of muscle is used, this will lead to ischemic necrosis, failure of reinnervation, and subsequent neuroma formation. Ischemic muscle grafts may also predispose to surgical site infection, which is particularly relevant in the population of patients receiving extremity amputations given their comorbidities. In addition, RPNI surgery has the risk of possible additional donor site pain from the harvest of free muscle grafts.

Specific limitations in TMR surgery include the frequent size discrepancy between the large residual donor nerve and smaller recipient motor nerve branch, which is a known factor for producing a neuroma-in-continuity.[36,37] However, some studies have shown that these neuromas-in-continuity have not been symptomatic.[38] Limitations to TMR surgery include the necessary transection of an otherwise uninjured motor nerve that has sensory and motor fibers, potentially increasing the risk of creating new neuromas. In addition, if there is no expendable target motor nerve branch readily available, then TMR surgery is not possible. In these cases, one proposed solution is to perform RPNI surgery.[44] Additionally, TMR-related denervation atrophy of donated muscle can be seen as a limitation.[45]

For both RPNI and TMR surgeries, failure in treating postamputation pain may also be secondary to "unmasking" as some patients have described their pain moving to a new nerve distribution area following neurectomy.[44,46] As such, an eventual revision surgery to address these other nerves is sometimes necessary.

PROSTHETIC USE: REGENERATIVE PERIPHERAL NERVE INTERFACE AND TARGETED MUSCLE REINNERVATION SURGERIES

Prosthetic rehabilitation after upper extremity amputation continues to evolve, and optimizing functional restoration following limb loss is essential. Achieving a high level of function with prosthetic limbs remains a significant challenge. For decades, the body-powered prosthesis was the dominant strategy. These devices use cables and a harness system to control a clasping hook, but the additive function is rudimentary and very limited. While these devices are still used and can meet basic functional needs ("helper hand"), they do not have nearly the function or intuitive control as the native arm or hand. More recently, myoelectric prosthetic devices are powered limbs that have the potential to better emulate the multiple functions of a human hand and arm,[47] but these robotic limbs require the input of motor command signals emanating from the residual limb. Both RPNI and TMR surgeries have the potential to enable capture of discrete motors commands to allow for discrete control of a neuroprosthetic device.

RPNI surgery has been used successfully for real-time prosthetic device control in patients with an upper extremity amputation.[48–50] With the RPNI technique, the formation of new neuromuscular junctions between the peripheral nerve and free skeletal muscle grafts allows for volitional neural signals to be transduced into large electromyographic (EMG) signals produced by the contracting RPNI muscle tissue. This not only obviates older strategies of placing electrodes directly onto the peripheral nerve, which led to iatrogenic injury and inevitable signal degradation, but also results in improved signal-to-noise ratios. In human trials, RPNI surgery was shown to transduce efferent motor actional potentials into large amplitude compound muscle actional potentials with very high signal-to-noise ratios that translate to high-fidelity prosthetic control of extrinsic and intrinsic hand and finger functions.[48] To increase signal specificity, larger nerves can be separated into multiple RPNIs so that the motor signals contained in one peripheral nerve can be spatially segregated and captured by multiple implanted electrodes. In this manner, RPNI surgery has the immense potential to facilitate multiple degrees of freedom in prosthetic movement. For example, human trials have shown independent signals from RPNIs corresponding flexion and extension of individual fingers, intrinsic thumb movements, wrist rotation, as well as coordinated simultaneous control of multiple movements.[48,50]

TMR surgery has also been used successfully for real-time prosthetic device control. TMR surgery can create individual motor points on a muscle with discernible EMG signals that can be detected by surface electrodes. By transferring multiple nerves, TMR myoelectric signals can allow intuitive, simultaneous control of multiple joints as compared to a single flexion and extension pair of muscles in conventional myoelectric control. With TMR surgery, patients typically have at least 4 total myoelectric control sites, 2 for the elbow and 2 for the hand, enabling natural and easier operation of a prosthesis. In addition, each signal is independently modulated and not jointly connected, which enables simultaneous control of the elbow and hand, overcoming the traditional mode switching that is necessary in conventional myoelectric control prosthesis. Various trials have shown that TMR surgery can yield good control of several prosthetic degrees of freedom with improved performance as compared with conventional myoelectric control.[51,52]

RPNI and TMR surgeries have many similarities when used in prosthetic rehabilitation. A key difference is that TMR surgery requires purposeful denervation of a local muscle prior to nerve transfer. This results in a spatial limitation as there may only be a finite number of motor nerves in a given area accessible for nerve transfer. Additionally, the prosthetic experience for TMR surgery has centered around the use of surface EMG electrodes, which have very different electrophysiologic capabilities as compared to the implanted electrodes that have been used for RPNI prosthetic experiments. Certainly, efforts that pair implantable electrode technology with TMR surgery would be expected to yield more discrete and reliable motor command signals to better control upper extremity prosthetic devices.

FUTURE DIRECTION

There is robust basic science and clinical research relating to both RPNI and TMR surgeries for the management of postamputation pain and for facilitating prosthetic control. Therefore, both modalities show significant promise in the rehabilitation of upper extremity amputation patients. Ultimately, an ideal prosthetic interface will also provide meaningful sensory feedback that serves to optimize complex movements of individual fingers, modulate the force produced by a robotic device, and augment prosthetic embodiment.

To improve sensory tactile feedback, including touch, pressure, proprioception for prosthetics, the dermal sensory regenerative peripheral nerve interface (DS-RPNI) was expanded from the RPNI concept. Instead of a free skeletal muscle graft, the DS-RPNI utilizes a free dermal graft secured to the end of a transected sensory nerve. Experimentally, this variation of the RPNI has shown promise in decreasing neuroma formation as well as allowing for restoration of tactile sensation to improve function in human prosthetics limbs.[53] As such, DS-RPNI may be an improved physiologic match for the prevention of sensory nerve neuromas, such as the superficial radial sensory nerve branch in upper extremity amputations. Additionally, to integrate sensory and motor signals, the composite RPNI (C-RPNI) has also been developed.[54] The C-RPNI combines free dermal and muscle graft around a sensorimotor nerve, and it has shown capability in transducing both sensory and motor action potentials in rodent models.[54] Additionally, targeted sensory reinnervation is an exploratory modification of TMR surgery that involves rerouting sensory axons to purposefully denervated areas of skin.[55] In all these methods, the ability to provide afferent signals back to the central nervous system not only improves prosthetic function but also serves to further reduce phantom limb pain in upper extremity amputation patients.[56,57]

SUMMARY

Upper extremity amputation is a devastating loss, and rehabilitation efforts should focus on mitigating postamputation pain and maximizing functional restoration. Both RPNI and TMR surgeries have shown efficacy in mitigating residual limb pain and phantom limb pain. In turn, both strategies can play a role in improving the quality of life after amputation and reducing the consumption of pain medications. From a prosthetic control standpoint, both RPNI and TMR surgeries capitalize on the physiologic process of muscle reinnervation to capture efferent motor commands from peripheral nerves, but there are some important differences between the 2 strategies in terms of technique and the potential number of prosthetic degrees of freedom. Consideration of these differences should be the central drivers when deciding which patient will best be served by either of these strategies. In select patients, optimal prosthetic rehabilitation may even involve the synergistic use of both RPNI and TMR surgeries.

CLINICS CARE POINTS

- RPNI and TMR surgeries can be used to mitigate neuroma development and treat residual limb pain and phantom limb pain.

- RPNI surgery can be performed on all peripheral nerves and interfascicular dissection is recommended for large caliber nerves to optimize the ratio of regenerating axons to free muscle graft fibers.

- RPNI muscle grafts should be harvested from healthy skeletal muscle without the use of cautery and be approximately 30 mm long × 20 mm wide × 5 mm thick.

- Avoid local or regional anesthetic during TMR surgery to facilitate the identification of potential motor nerves with a handheld nerve stimulator.

- For a given level of upper extremity amputation, the nerve transfers involved in TMR surgery can be variable. Additionally, there may be a limited number of motor branches that will be purposefully sacrificed during TMR surgery. For this reason, nerve transfers involving functionally important nerves (eg, median nerve, and ulnar nerve) should be prioritized over others.

DISCLOSURE

T.A. Kung is the chief medical officer and cofounder of Blue Arbor Technologies, Inc, a prosthetics interface company. Otherwise, the authors have no commercial or financial conflicts of interest or any other funding sources related to this study.

REFERENCES

1. Owings MF, Kozak LJ. Ambulatory and inpatient procedures in the United States. Vital Health Stat 1996; 13(139):1–119.

2. Chalya PL, Mabula JB, Dass RM, et al. Major limb amputations: a tertiary hospital experience in northwestern Tanzania. J Orthop Surg Res 2012;7:18.

3. Ziegler-Graham K, MacKenzie EJ, Ephraim PL, et al. Estimating the prevalence of limb loss in the United States: 2005 to 2050. Arch Phys Med Rehabil 2008; 89(3):422–9.

4. Ephraim PL, Wegener ST, MacKenzie EJ, et al. Phantom pain, residual limb pain, and back pain in amputees: results of a national survey. Arch Phys Med Rehabil 2005;86(10):1910–9.

5. Ehde DM, Czerniecki JM, Smith DG, et al. Chronic phantom sensations, phantom pain, residual limb pain, and other regional pain after lower limb amputation. Arch Phys Med Rehabil 2000;81(8): 1039–44.

6. Smith DG, Ehde DM, Legro MW, et al. Phantom limb, residual limb, and back pain after lower extremity amputations. Clin Orthop Relat Res 1999;(361): 29–38.

7. Hsu E, Cohen SP. Postamputation pain: epidemiology, mechanisms, and treatment. J Pain Res 2013;6:121–36.

8. Lans J, Hoftiezer Y, Lozano-Calderón SA, et al. Risk factors for neuropathic pain following major upper extremity amputation. J Reconstr Microsurg 2021; 37(5):413–20.

9. Menorca RM, Fussell TS, Elfar JC. Nerve physiology: mechanisms of injury and recovery. Hand Clin 2013; 29(3):317–30.

10. Soroush M, Modirian E, Masoumi M. Neuroma in bilateral upper limb amputation. Orthopedics 2008; 31(12).

11. Geraghty TJ, Jones LE. Painful neuromata following upper limb amputation. Prosthet Orthot Int 1996; 20(3):176–81.

12. Buchheit T, Van de Ven T, Hsia HL, et al. Pain phenotypes and associated clinical risk factors following traumatic amputation: results from Veterans Integrated Pain Evaluation Research (VIPER). Pain Med 2016;17(1):149–61.

13. Hanley MA, Ehde DM, Jensen M, et al. Chronic pain associated with upper-limb loss. Am J Phys Med Rehabil 2009;88(9):742–51 [quiz 752, 779].

14. Sehirlioglu A, Ozturk C, Yazicioglu K, et al. Painful neuroma requiring surgical excision after lower limb amputation caused by landmine explosions. Int Orthop 2009;33(2):533–6.

15. Dellon AL, Mackinnon SE. Treatment of the painful neuroma by neuroma resection and muscle implantation. Plast Reconstr Surg 1986;77(3):427–38.

16. Ducic I, Mesbahi AN, Attinger CE, et al. The role of peripheral nerve surgery in the treatment of chronic pain associated with amputation stumps. Plast Reconstr Surg 2008;121(3):908–14.

17. Burchiel KJ, Johans TJ, Ochoa J. The surgical treatment of painful traumatic neuromas. J Neurosurg 1993;78(5):714–9.

18. Robbins TH. Nerve capping in the treatment of troublesome terminal neuromata. Br J Plast Surg 1986; 39(2):239–40.

19. Pet MA, Ko JH, Friedly JL, et al. Does targeted nerve implantation reduce neuroma pain in amputees? Clin Orthop Relat Res 2014;472(10):2991–3001.

20. Hung YH, Wu CH, Özçakar L, et al. Ultrasound-guided steroid injections for two painful neuromas in the stump of a below-elbow amputee. Am J Phys Med Rehabil 2016;95(5):e73–4.

21. Soin A, Fang ZP, Velasco J. Peripheral neuromodulation to treat postamputation pain. Prog Neurol Surg 2015;29:158–67.

22. White TP, Devor ST. Skeletal muscle regeneration and plasticity of grafts. Exerc Sport Sci Rev 1993; 21:263–95.

23. Dumont NA, Bentzinger CF, Sincennes MC, et al. Satellite cells and skeletal muscle regeneration. Compr Physiol 2015;5(3):1027–59.

24. Bader D. Reinnervation of motor endplate-containing and motor endplate-less muscle grafts. Dev Biol 1980;77(2):315–27.

25. Kung TA, Bueno RA, Alkhalefah GK, et al. Innovations in prosthetic interfaces for the upper extremity. Plast Reconstr Surg 2013;132(6):1515–23.

26. Langhals NB, Woo SL, Moon JD, et al. Electrically stimulated signals from a long-term regenerative peripheral nerve interface. Annu Int Conf IEEE Eng Med Biol Soc 2014;2014:1989–92.

27. Woo SL, Kung TA, Brown DL, et al. Regenerative peripheral nerve interfaces for the treatment of postamputation neuroma pain: a pilot study. Plast Reconstr Surg Glob Open 2016;4(12):e1038.

28. Kubiak CA, Kemp SWP, Cederna PS, et al. Prophylactic regenerative peripheral nerve interfaces to prevent postamputation pain. Plast Reconstr Surg 2019;144(3):421e–30e.

29. Hijjawi JB, Kuiken TA, Lipschutz RD, et al. Improved myoelectric prosthesis control accomplished using multiple nerve transfers. Plast Reconstr Surg 2006; 118(7):1573–8.

30. Kuiken TA, Dumanian GA, Lipschutz RD, et al. The use of targeted muscle reinnervation for improved myoelectric prosthesis control in a bilateral shoulder disarticulation amputee. Prosthet Orthot Int 2004; 28(3):245–53.

31. Kuiken T. Targeted reinnervation for improved prosthetic function. Phys Med Rehabil Clin 2006;17(1):1–13.

32. Henderson JT, Koenig ZA, Climov M, et al. Targeted muscle reinnervation: a systematic review of nerve transfers for the upper extremity. Ann Plast Surg 2023;90(5):462–70.

33. Kuiken TA, Barlow AK, Hargrove L, et al. Targeted muscle reinnervation for the upper and lower extremity. Tech Orthop 2017;32(2):109–16.

34. Janes LE, Fracol ME, Dumanian GA, et al. Targeted muscle reinnervation for the treatment of neuroma. Hand Clin 2021;37(3):345–59.

35. Valerio IL, Dumanian GA, Jordan SW, et al. Preemptive treatment of phantom and residual limb pain with targeted muscle reinnervation at the time of major limb amputation. J Am Coll Surg 2019;228(3): 217–26.

36. Valerio I, Schulz SA, West J, et al. Targeted muscle reinnervation combined with a vascularized pedicled regenerative peripheral nerve interface. Plast Reconstr Surg Glob Open 2020;8(3):e2689.

37. Mavrogenis AF, Pavlakis K, Stamatoukou A, et al. Current treatment concepts for neuromas-in-continuity. Injury 2008;39(Suppl 3):S43–8.

38. Dumanian GA, Potter BK, Mioton LM, et al. Targeted muscle reinnervation treats neuroma and phantom pain in major limb amputees: a randomized clinical trial. Ann Surg 2019;270(2):238–46.

39. Kurlander DE, Wee C, Chepla KJ, et al. TMRpni: combining two peripheral nerve management techniques. Plast Reconstr Surg Glob Open 2020; 8(10):e3132.

40. Souza JM, Cheesborough JE, Ko JH, et al. Targeted muscle reinnervation: a novel approach to postamputation neuroma pain. Clin Orthop Relat Res 2014;472(10):2984–90.

41. O'Brien AL, Jordan SW, West JM, et al. Targeted muscle reinnervation at the time of upper-extremity amputation for the treatment of pain severity and symptoms. J Hand Surg Am 2021;46(1):72.e1–10.

42. Goodyear EG, O'Brien AL, West JM, et al. Targeted muscle reinnervation at the time of amputation decreases recurrent symptomatic neuroma formation. Plast Reconstr Surg 2023. https://doi.org/10.1097/PRS.0000000000010692.

43. Morag Y, Ganesh Kumar N, Hamill JB, et al. Ultrasound appearance of regenerative peripheral nerve interface with clinical correlation. Skeletal Radiol 2023;52(6):1137–57.

44. Hoyt BW, Potter BK, Souza JM. Nerve interface strategies for neuroma management and prevention: a conceptual approach guided by institutional experience. Hand Clin 2021;37(3):373–82.

45. Lineaweaver WC, Zhang F. Clarifying the role of targeted muscle reinnervation in amputation management. J Am Coll Surg 2019;229(6):635.

46. Gomez-Rexrode AE, Kennedy SH, Brown DL. Unmasked neuropathic pain after neurectomy: a case series and review of the literature. Plast Reconstr Surg Glob Open 2023;11(8):e5221.

47. Østlie K, Lesjø IM, Franklin RJ, et al. Prosthesis use in adult acquired major upper-limb amputees: patterns of wear, prosthetic skills and the actual use of prostheses in activities of daily life. Disabil Rehabil Assist Technol 2012;7(6):479–93.

48. Vu PP, Vaskov AK, Irwin ZT, et al. A regenerative peripheral nerve interface allows real-time control of an artificial hand in upper limb amputees. Sci Transl Med 2020;12(533).

49. Ortiz-Catalan M, Mastinu E, Sassu P, et al. Self-contained neuromusculoskeletal arm prostheses. N Engl J Med 2020;382(18):1732–8.

50. Ortiz-Catalan M, Zbinden J, Millenaar J, et al. A highly integrated bionic hand with neural control

and feedback for use in daily life. Sci Robot 2023; 8(83):eadf7360.

51. Hargrove LJ, Lock BA, Simon AM. Pattern recognition control outperforms conventional myoelectric control in upper limb patients with targeted muscle reinnervation. Annu Int Conf IEEE Eng Med Biol Soc 2013;2013:1599–602.

52. Kuiken TA, Li G, Lock BA, et al. Targeted muscle reinnervation for real-time myoelectric control of multifunction artificial arms. JAMA 2009;301(6): 619–28.

53. Sando IC, Adidharma W, Nedic A, et al. Dermal sensory regenerative peripheral nerve interface for re-establishing sensory nerve feedback in peripheral afferents in the rat. Plast Reconstr Surg 2023; 151(5):804e–13e.

54. Svientek SR, Ursu DC, Cederna PS, et al. Fabrication of the composite regenerative peripheral nerve interface (C-RPNI) in the adult rat. J Vis Exp 2020;156.

55. Gardetto A, Baur EM, Prahm C, et al. Reduction of phantom limb pain and improved proprioception through a TSR-based surgical technique: a case series of four patients with lower limb amputation. J Clin Med 2021;10(17).

56. Hebert JS, Olson JL, Morhart MJ, et al. Novel targeted sensory reinnervation technique to restore functional hand sensation after transhumeral amputation. IEEE Trans Neural Syst Rehabil Eng 2014; 22(4):765–73.

57. Hebert JS, Chan KM, Dawson MR. Cutaneous sensory outcomes from three transhumeral targeted reinnervation cases. Prosthet Orthot Int 2016;40(3): 303–10.

UNITED STATES POSTAL SERVICE® Statement of Ownership, Management, and Circulation (All Periodicals Publications Except Requester Publications)

1. Publication Title	2. Publication Number	3. Filing Date
CLINICS IN PLASTIC SURGERY	006 – 530	9/18/2024

4. Issue Frequency	5. Number of Issues Published Annually	6. Annual Subscription Price
JAN, APR, JUL,OCT	4	$576.00

7. Complete Mailing Address of Known Office of Publication (Not printer) (Street, city, county, state, and ZIP+4®)

ELSEVIER INC.
230 Park Avenue, Suite 800
New York, NY 10169

Contact Person
Malathi Samayan
Telephone (Include area code)
91-44-4299-4507

8. Complete Mailing Address of Headquarters or General Business Office of Publisher (Not printer)

ELSEVIER INC.
230 Park Avenue, Suite 800
New York, NY 10169

9. Full Names and Complete Mailing Addresses of Publisher, Editor, and Managing Editor (Do not leave blank)

Publisher (Name and complete mailing address)

Dolores Meloni, ELSEVIER INC.
1600 JOHN F KENNEDY BLVD. SUITE 1600
PHILADELPHIA, PA 19103-2899

Editor (Name and complete mailing address)

Stacy Eastman, ELSEVIER INC.
1600 JOHN F KENNEDY BLVD. SUITE 1600
PHILADELPHIA, PA 19103-2899

Managing Editor (Name and complete mailing address)

PATRICK MANLEY, ELSEVIER INC.
1600 JOHN F KENNEDY BLVD. SUITE 1600
PHILADELPHIA, PA 19103-2899

10. Owner (Do not leave blank. If the publication is owned by a corporation, give the name and address of the corporation immediately followed by the names and addresses of all stockholders owning or holding 1 percent or more of the total amount of stock. If not owned by a corporation, give the names and addresses of the individual owners. If owned by a partnership or other unincorporated firm, give its name and address as well as those of each individual owner. If the publication is published by a nonprofit organization, give its name and address.)

Full Name	Complete Mailing Address
WHOLLY OWNED SUBSIDIARY OF REED/ELSEVIER, US HOLDINGS	1600 JOHN F KENNEDY BLVD. SUITE 1600 PHILADELPHIA, PA 19103-2899

11. Known Bondholders, Mortgagees, and Other Security Holders Owning or Holding 1 Percent or More of Total Amount of Bonds, Mortgages, or Other Securities. If none, check box ▶ ☐ None

Full Name	Complete Mailing Address
N/A	

12. Tax Status (For completion by nonprofit organizations authorized to mail at nonprofit rates) (Check one)
The purpose, function, and nonprofit status of this organization and the exempt status for federal income tax purposes:
☒ Has Not Changed During Preceding 12 Months
☐ Has Changed During Preceding 12 Months (Publisher must submit explanation of change with this statement)

PS Form **3526**, July 2014 [Page 1 of 4 (see instructions page 4)] PSN: 7530-01-000-9931 PRIVACY NOTICE: See our privacy policy on www.usps.com.

13. Publication Title	14. Issue Date for Circulation Data Below
CLINICS IN PLASTIC SURGERY	AUGUST 2024

15. Extent and Nature of Circulation			Average No. Copies Each Issue During Preceding 12 Months	No. Copies of Single Issue Published Nearest to Filing Date
a. Total Number of Copies (Net press run)			268	235
b. Paid Circulation (By Mail and Outside the Mail)	(1)	Mailed Outside-County Paid Subscriptions Stated on PS Form 3541 (Include paid distribution above nominal rate, advertiser's proof copies, and exchange copies)	131	116
	(2)	Mailed In-County Paid Subscriptions Stated on PS Form 3541 (Include paid distribution above nominal rate, advertiser's proof copies, and exchange copies)	0	0
	(3)	Paid Distribution Outside the Mails Including Sales Through Dealers and Carriers, Street Vendors, Counter Sales, and Other Paid Distribution Outside USPS®	83	73
	(4)	Paid Distribution by Other Classes of Mail Through the USPS (e.g. First-Class Mail®)	0	0
c. Total Paid Distribution (Sum of 15b (1), (2), (3), and (4))		▶	214	189
d. Free or Nominal Rate Distribution (By Mail and Outside the Mail)	(1)	Free or Nominal Rate Outside-County Copies included on PS Form 3541	33	25
	(2)	Free or Nominal Rate In-County Copies Included on PS Form 3541	0	0
	(3)	Free or Nominal Rate Copies Mailed at Other Classes Through the USPS (e.g. First-Class Mail)	0	0
	(4)	Free or Nominal Rate Distribution Outside the Mail (Carriers or other means)	0	0
e. Total Free or Nominal Rate Distribution (Sum of 15d (1), (2), (3) and (4))		▶	33	25
f. Total Distribution (Sum of 15c and 15e)		▶	247	214
g. Copies not Distributed (See Instructions to Publishers #4 (page #3))		▶	21	21
h. Total (Sum of 15f and g)		▶	268	235
i. Percent Paid (15c divided by 15f times 100)		▶	86.63%	88.31%

* If you are claiming electronic copies, go to line 16 on page 3. If you are not claiming electronic copies, skip to line 17 on page 3.

PS Form **3526**, July 2014 (Page 2 of 4)

16. Electronic Copy Circulation	Average No. Copies Each Issue During Preceding 12 Months	No. Copies of Single Issue Published Nearest to Filing Date
a. Paid Electronic Copies	▶	
b. Total Paid Print Copies (Line 15c) + Paid Electronic Copies (Line 16a)	▶	
c. Total Print Distribution (Line 15f) + Paid Electronic Copies (Line 16a)	▶	
d. Percent Paid (Both Print & Electronic Copies) (16b divided by 16c × 100)	▶	

☒ I certify that 50% of all my distributed copies (electronic and print) are paid above a nominal price.

17. Publication of Statement of Ownership

☒ If the publication is a general publication, publication of this statement is required. Will be printed in the October 2024 issue of this publication. ☐ Publication not required.

18. Signature and Title of Editor, Publisher, Business Manager, or Owner

Malathi Samayan — Distribution Controller

Malathi Samayan - Distribution Controller

Date 9/18/2024

I certify that all information furnished on this form is true and complete. I understand that anyone who furnishes false or misleading information on this form or who omits material or information requested on the form may be subject to criminal sanctions (including fines and imprisonment) and/or civil sanctions (including civil penalties).

PS Form **3526**, July 2014 (Page 3 of 4)

PRIVACY NOTICE: See our privacy policy on www.usps.com.

Printed and bound by CPI Group (UK) Ltd, Croydon, CR0 4YY

08/05/2025

01864748-0018